MANUAL OF ELECTRONEUROMYOGRAPHY

manual of
ELECTRONEUROMYOGRAPHY
second edition

HYMAN L. COHEN, M.D.

Clinical Assistant Professor of Neurology, Department of Neurology, Loyola University of Chicago, Chicago, Illinois; Attending Physician and Medical Director, Department of Electrodiagnostics, Methodist Hospital, Gary, Indiana

JOEL BRUMLIK, M.D., Ph.D.

Professor and Chairman, Department of Neurology, Loyola University of Chicago, Chicago; Attending Physician, Department of Neurology, Foster G. McGaw Hospital, Maywood, Illinois

Medical Department
HARPER & ROW, PUBLISHERS
Hagerstown, Maryland
New York, San Francisco, London

76–77–78–79–80–81—10–9–8–7–6–5–4–3–2–1

Cover and text designed by Pamela M. Lichtenstein

Library of Congress Cataloging in Publication Data

Cohen, Hyman L
    Manual of electroneuromyography.

    Includes bibliographical references and index.
    1. Electromyography. I. Brumlik, Joel, joint author.
II. Title.
RC77.5.C6 1976   616.8   76–17578
ISBN 0–06–140644–9

CONTENTS

CASE PRESENTATIONS

PREFACE

The second edition of this manual endeavors, as did the first, to instruct medical students, house staff, and graduate physicians in the practical elements of nerve and muscle testing by means of electrophysiology. In a direct, pragmatic manner, it allows the beginning student at any professional level to gain expertise in the actual performance of tests, to interpret the results in the context of the clinical findings, and to report the findings in a clear concise manner. This edition incorporates details about currently available equipment, new information on technique, and additional case reports of pertinent disorders. There are many new illustrations, including photographs of the NCV studies. The problem solving exercises have been expanded, and additional references have been included throughout.

The introduction orients the beginning student to the study of ENM. Chapter 1 describes the essential features that many available commercial ENM units have in common. Chapters 2–4 describe the techniques of NSS, EMG, and EDX, respectively, as listed in the table. In each of these chapters, a general description of the components of each unit and definition of terms (1) and parameters is followed by a step-by-step description of each technique with emphasis on actual performance of the procedure. Following this is a discussion of the artifacts and sources of error attendant to the specific technique. Normal and abnormal findings with representative clinical correlations are then presented. Finally, the steps to be followed by the examiner are summarized in detail. Frequent references are made throughout the text to figures which illustrate the actual operation of the equipment. Chapter 5 is devoted to case reports in which these techniques are used to solve clinical problems. "Unknowns" are provided for the student to solve.

Adhering to a format of simplicity, clarity, and brevity, we have designed this manual as a cornerstone upon which the physician can expand his knowledge and techniques; this manual is not for the advanced electroneuromyographer. Since the publication of the first edition, several excellent texts have become available, to which we refer in appropriate chapters. Techniques of a special nature (such as *in vitro* intracellular microelectrode recordings) and research procedures which are not yet applicable to commonly encountered clinical situations will be referred to by appropriate source material.

This manual, then, is a guide to the steps necessary to perform the tests collec-

MAJOR STUDIES PERFORMED IN ENM

Nerve stimulation studies (NSS)	Electromyography (EMG)	Electrodiagnosis (EDX)

1. Nerve conduction velocity (NCV)
  a. Motor
  b. Sensory
2. Nerve segment conduction
3. Latency
4. Compound muscle action potential
5. Repetitive stimulation studies
6. Reflex studies
	1. Motor unit potentials (MUP)
	  a. Parameters of individual MUPs
	  b. Contraction characteristics
	  c. Single fiber potentials
	2. Insertion potentials
	3. Spontaneous potentials
	  a. Fibrillations
	  b. Fasciculations
	  c. Bizarre high frequency potentials (BHFP)
	  d. Myotonic discharges
		1. Chronaxie
		2. Rheobase
		3. Strength-Duration (S-D curve)
		4. Repetitive stimulus (R-S curve)
		5. Galvanic tetanus ratio (GTR)

tively referred to as electroneuromyography (ENM): NSS, EMG, and EDX. Confusion arises over the term EMG, which has been used to refer both to needle electrode studies of muscle as well as to all ENM studies. The term ENM was used by Carpendale (2), and we suggest that it is an appropriate term to encompass all studies in this field: NSS, EMG, and EDX.

Our intent is that this manual will help students and physicians in practice apply ENM in various branches of medicine, including such diverse fields as general surgery, internal medicine, neurology, neurosurgery, orthopedics, otorhinolaryngology, physiatry, and psychiatry.

H. L. C.
J. B.

REFERENCES

1. Terminology of Electromyography. Bull Am Assoc EMG EDX, 1967
2. Carpendale M: The localization of ulnar nerve compression in the hand and arm; an improved method of Electroneuromyography. Arch Phys Med Rehabil 47: 325–330, 1967

ACKNOWLEDGMENTS

The authors extend their appreciation to all their colleagues whose special talents aided us in producing this book. We also are grateful for permission to publish the case histories of patients referred by Dr. Benjamin Boshes, the late Dr. Roland Mackay, Dr. Ogelvie Paul, Dr. David Drachman, Dr. William Kernohan, and Dr. Howard Alt. We are most appreciative of the assistance rendered by Dr. Emanual Ross (neuropathology), Dr. Enricque Palacios (neuroradiology), and the Department of Photography and Medical Illustration of Loyola University Medical Center (Ms. Margaret Conneely, Ms. Margot Snyder, Dr. Tony Marchese and Ms. Peggy Martino).

We are grateful to those who have presented us with constructive comments regarding the first edition and express our gratitude to Ms. Patricia Salinas and Ms. Mary Bresolin for preparing the manuscript.

This edition is dedicated with deep affection to our families.

INTRODUCTION

Electroneuromyography (ENM) is a well-established technique for determining the functional integrity of the lower motor neuron (anterior horn cell and its axon), neuromyal junction, muscle, peripheral sensory apparatus, and some reflex pathways. The electroneuromyographer must learn the capabilities and limitations of the technique and the reasonable interpretation of the results.

The several areas fundamental to ENM in which the electroneuromyographer must be competent include 1) anatomy, physiology, and pathology of the nervous system, with emphasis on nerve and muscle; 2) medical electronics, with detailed understanding of the specific instrumentation used, including safety regulations; and 3) clinical neurology and physiatry related to the disorders encountered in the ENM laboratory.

The following should be available in the laboratory: at least one anatomy text, with details of the location and relationships of muscles and nerves (6, 9, 20, 21, 24, 28); one text on functional neuroanatomy, especially with reference to the peripheral nervous system (12, 27); a text on examination of nerves and muscles (2, 12, 29); a text on nerve and muscle pathology (1, 4, 7, 8, 11, 27, 29); a general textbook of neurology (2, 17); and a detailed instruction and trouble-shooting manual on the equipment (10, 25). Texts which the authors have found useful in their laboratories are listed in the references (1–30).

Each patient referred to the laboratory should bring some type of requisition with him so that the examiner understands the reason for the referral (this record can be sent in advance of the patient if circumstances so allow). After reading the material from the referring source, the examiner should confirm this information with the patient, ask further questions, and perform an appropriate examination; when the patient's history and physical findings are not available, the electroneuromyographer must perform a more complete neurologic examination. A request to examine only certain nerves and muscles by ENM should not preclude further testing. As with most studies, the more diligent the search the more fruitful the results.

Each unit of ENM–nerve stimulation studies (NSS), electromyography (EMG), and electrodiagnosis (EDX)–will find application, depending on the clinical problem at hand. For example, in a patient with a *peripheral neuropathy,* NSS may yield the most significant information. It may indicate a mononeuropathy, mononeuritis multiplex, or a widespread neuropathy. These studies may localize a single site as the defect in the system, such as an ulnar neuropathy at the elbow. This may lead the clinician to a diagnosis of an entrapment neuropathy, an infectious process, or some other etiology. Analysis of the compound-muscle-action potential provides information about the nature of the defect: In primary axonal lesions, the amplitude of the evoked response is markedly diminished; whereas, in lesions which primarily affect the myelin sheath, not only is the conduction velocity slowed, but the duration of the compound-muscle-action potential is prolonged.

In a patient with *amyotrophic lateral sclerosis,* EMG will be the most informative of the three techniques. Early in the disease, nerve conduction velocity (NCV) values are normal but, at the same time, needle electrode examination reveals evidence of denervation in a widespread pattern, with fasciculations and changes in the motor units.

In a patient recovering from a traumatic lesion of a peripheral nerve, EDX may be most useful in monitoring the course of recovery. Through this technique, signs of recovery may be detected earlier than by needle electrode exploration of muscles or by NSS. Electroneuromyography thus will provide information when diseases affect the anterior horn cell, peripheral nerve (sensory and motor), myoneural junction, and muscle.

A single examination may not be adequate. Serial studies may be required both for patient comfort and to follow the course of disease. This should be indicated to the referring physician in the report. Judgment always is required to obtain the maximum information from a given patient. For example, abnormal findings elicited in one extremity should prompt the examiner to search for involvement in other areas. The study requires a knowledge of basic clinical neurology and suspicion on the part of the examiner. On the other hand, to exhaust the patient with endless studies of any kind is unnecessary. A balance must exist between too brief a test and too extensive an examination which tires the patient and adds little to the diagnosis.

With these concepts in mind, the electroneuromyographer is responsible for at least three functions in the laboratory:

1. Perform a thorough, reliable, reasonably efficient, and pertinent study.
2. Locate the site of pathology, assess its degree and, if possible, its nature.
3. Report the findings in a manner which is understandable, with appropriate documentation useful for diagnosis and therapy.

REFERENCES

1. Adams RD, Denny-Brown D, Pearson CM: Diseases of Muscle, 2nd ed. Hagerstown, Hoeber, Harper & Row, 1962, p 735
2. Baker AB, Baker LH (eds): Clinical Neurology. New York, Harper & Row, 1974, p 3 Vols
3. Bendall JR: Muscles, Molecules and Movement. New York, American Elsevier, 1969, p 219
3a. Berlin HM: Danger Lurks! QST:15–17, 1976
4. Bethlem J: Muscle Pathology. New York, American Elsevier, 1970, pp 132

5. Brazier M: The Electrical Activity of the Nervous System, 3rd ed. New York, Macmillan, 1968, p 317
6. Delagi EF, Perotto A, Iazzetti J, Morrison D: Anatomic Guide for the Electromyographer. The Limbs. Springfield, Ill, CC Thomas, 1975, p 207
7. Dyck PJ, Thomas PK, Lambert EH (eds): Peripheral Neuropathy. Philadelphia, WB Saunders, 1975, p 1438
8. Escourolle R, Porier J: Manual of Basic Neuropathology. Philadelphia, WB Saunders, 1973, p 209
9. Goodgold J: Anatomical Correlates of Clinical Electromyography. Baltimore, William & Wilkins, 1974, p 153
10. Grass E, Grass A: Electrical Safety. Quincy, MA, Grass Instruments, 1972, p 25
11. Greenfield JG, Shy GM, Alvord EC, Berg L: An Atlas of Muscle Pathology in Neuromuscular Diseases. London, E&S Livingstone, 1957, p 104
12. WB Saunders, 1953, pp 333
13. Hubbard JI, Llinas R, Quastel EMJ: Electrophysiological Analysis of Synaptic Transmission. Baltimore, Williams & Wilkins, 1969, p 372
14. Katz B: Nerve, Muscle and Synapse. New York McGraw–Hill, 1966, p 193
15. Katz B: The Release of Neural Transmitter Substances. Springfield, Ill, CC Thomas, 1969, pp 60
16. McLennan H: Synaptic Transmission, 2nd ed. Philadelphia, WB Saunders, 1970, p 134
17. Merritt H: Textbook of Neurology. Philadelphia, Lea & Febiger, 1973, pp 844
18. Offner FF: Electronics for Biologists. New York, McGraw–Hill, 1967, p 185
19. Pinelli P, Buchthal F, Thiebaut F (eds): Progress in Electromyography. Electroencephalogy Clin Neurophysiol [Suppl 22] Elsevier, 1962, p 184
20. Riddoch G (Chairman): Aids to the Investigation of Peripheral Nerve Injuries. London, His Majesty's Stationery Office, 1942, p 49
21. Romanes GJ (ed): Cunningham's Textbook of Anatomy, 10th ed. London Oxford University Press, 1964, p 1014
22. Ruch TC, Patton HD, Woodbury JW, Tower AL: Neurophysiology II, 2nd ed. Philadelphia, WB Saunders, 1965, pp 26–152
23. Safe Use of Electricity in Hospitals (Bull 76 BM). National Fire Protection Association 60 Batterymarch St, Boston, MA 02110
24. Spalteholtz W: Hand Atlas of Anatomy. Philadelphia, JB Lippincott, 1952, p 900
25. Starmer F, McIntosh H, Whalen R: Electrical hazards and cardiovascular function. N Engl J Med 284:181–186, 1971
26. Strong P: Biophysical Measurements. Beaverton, Oregon, Tektronix, 1970, p 499
27. Sunderland S: Nerves and Nerve Injuries. London, E&S Livingstone, 1968, p 1161
28. Truex RC, Carpenter MB: Human Neuroanatomy, 6th ed. Baltimore, Williams & Wilkins, 1969, p 673
29. Walton JN: Disorders of Voluntary Muscle, 3rd ed. Edinburgh & London, Churchill Livingstone, p 1149
30. Whitfield IC: An Introduction to Electronics for Physiological Workers, 2nd ed. New York, Macmillan, 1960, p 263

MANUAL OF ELECTRONEUROMYOGRAPHY

one

THE ENM LABORATORY

To assess the integrity of the peripheral nervous apparatus, ENM utilizes a variety of equipment which can be divided into four categories: 1) the nerve stimulation unit for NSS; 2) the EMG unit with needle electrodes for muscle examination; 3) the EDX unit; and 4) units for data display, storage, and analysis. Figure 1–1 is a view of an ENM laboratory with the various units identified.

Many commercial ENM units are available for clinical use. Indeed, some laboratories prefer to assemble units to meet their own special needs and specifications. The particulars of operations may vary from one unit to another, but the general principles outlined in this manual are common to all. When such equipment is purchased, one should bear in mind the nature of the studies to be performed (for example, whether the equipment will be used primarily for research or primarily for clinical purposes).

Before using the equipment, the electroneuromyographer should familiarize himself thoroughly with the manual of operation supplied with the unit. Modern electronic equipment is sophisticated and delicate. It should be handled carefully to ensure good function and long life. The preventative maintenance, recommended by the manufacturer should be performed at regular intervals. Needle electrodes should be checked regularly with a volt-ohmmeter for defects. The safety precautions for all electronic equipment also apply to ENM (5). Current leakage should be checked periodically by a qualified person.

The ENM laboratory has several requirements. Space should be sufficient to house the equipment, and an examining table, preferably made of wood, should be available. The room should be large enough to allow the electroneuromyographer and/or technician to work comfortably with the patient. The entrance to the room should be wide enough to allow carts as well as wheelchairs to enter. Space for data analysis and storage for both supplies and records must be available. A 10 × 12 ft (approximately 3 × 4 m) is a minimum space allocation for the main room.

The area requires controls for temperature because nerve conduction is affected by the temperature of the extremity (see Artifacts and Sources of Error, Ch. 2). A device to measure skin temperature is needed. A heat source should be available to warm a cool extremity. Most modern equipment need not be placed in a shielded

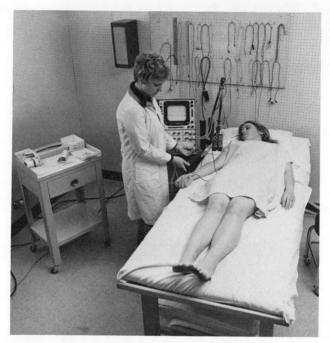

Fig. 1–1. Overall view of the ENM laboratory. Illustrated are the ENM machine, wooden table, a movable cart for accessories, and a peg board for convenient arrangement of stimulating and recording electrodes. An auxillary speaker is mounted on the wall to the left of the examiner.

room: Adequate grounding can eliminate extraneous signals. A rheostat (dimmer) control for room lighting is helpful for viewing oscilloscope displays. Reference texts and charts for nerve and muscle anatomy should be available (Introduction); many laboratories prefer to have such charts displayed for convenient reference (muscles, nerves, motor points and tables of normal ENM data). Laboratories which deal with the general medical population should have resuscitation equipment available for immediate use.

NERVE STIMULATION UNIT

The equipment for nerve stimulation studies includes an electronic stimulator which can deliver single or multiple monophasic, square-wave pulses of 0.05–2.0 msec in duration, with an intensity variable up to approximately 250 V. The distance between stimulating electrodes usually is fixed at 2.5–3.0 cm for surface stimulation. Surface electrodes used in NSS are illustrated in Figure 1–2. When needle electrodes are used for stimulation, they are placed adjacent to the nerve and this distance may be varied (2). The controls (for current strength, duration of pulse, repetitive stimulation, etc.) should be situated for ease of adjustment during the study. For convenience, the polarity of the stimulating electrodes should

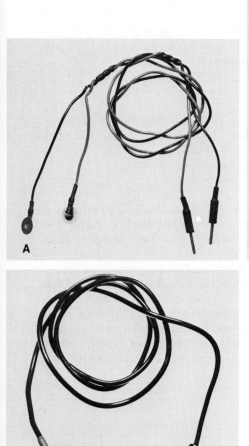

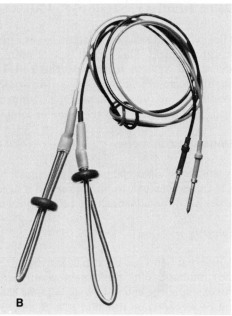

Fig. 1–2. Surface electrodes. A. Disc recording electrodes. B. Digit electrodes (for sensory recording or stimulating). C. Large disc electrode (for ground or indifferent).

be easily reversible (Artifacts and Sources of Error, Reversal of Polarity, and Fig. 2–21, Ch. 2). The equipment includes a preamplifier (for signal amplication) and an oscilloscope (for signal display). The unit contains a calibration signal (a known voltage/cm that can be displayed on the oscilloscope screen as a reference amplitude) and an accurate and precise time base.

DATA DISPLAY, STORAGE, AND ANALYSIS

The oscilloscope display of responses is rapid and vanishes before a detailed analysis can be made. Thus, some type of more permanent display is necessary. There are several ways to accomplish this end: 1) a storage oscilloscope; 2) a Polaroid Land camera; 3) light-sensitive (ultraviolet fiber optic) photographic paper; 4) sparkwriter on metallic paper; 5) a 35-mm or motion picture camera; and 6) a tape recorder for replay into the same or another system.

Storage Oscilloscope

A storage oscilloscope permits the signal to be viewed directly and immediately. The traces then can be photographed if needed. This method and direct recording paper have the advantage of prompt viewing.

Cameras

A Polaroid Land camera can be synchronized with both the oscilloscope sweep and the stimulator. With this camera, a number of traces can be placed on one picture. For example, the calibration signal, time base and the results of two or more stimuli can be recorded on one film (Ch. 3, Fig. 3–20).

The 35-mm still and motion picture cameras have a disadvantage: The results are not available until the film has been developed. Some units contain a mechanical dial calibrated in milliseconds and coupled to the oscilloscope trace, which moves a marker across the screen. When the latter is aligned with the onset of the evoked response, the latency (in milliseconds) can be read directly from the dial. This method has the disadvantages of providing no permanent record and no means of analyzing the compound-muscle-action potential. The apparatus also requires periodic calibration.

ELECTRONEUROMYOGRAPHIC UNIT

Audio System

The examiner must both *see* and *hear* the electrical activity emanating from the tissues. Both the visual and auditory displays are necessary so that small changes in amplitude can be seen on the oscilloscope, while the duration and frequency, which are best discerned by the ear, can be heard through the loudspeaker. Thus, an audio system is required which can reproduce sounds accurately from the frequency range of the amplifier. The amplifier frequency response should be flat between 2–10,000 Hz. The fidelity of the reproduction should be sufficient to distinguish the characteristic sounds of different potentials.

The alternative to this "hear and see" method is to record all potentials in some graphic form and to analyze them visually. This method consumes much more time but has the advantage of allowing the examiner to count the number of various types of potentials and thereby have access to a quantitative estimation of greater accuracy. Computer analysis of the potentials is a third alternative. This procedure is currently being developed.

Permanent Records

The storage of permanent records and redisplay methods described earlier are used both in NSSs and in EMG for one or several potentials. For longer periods of recording, the responses are most efficiently and economically placed on magnetic tape (Ch. 3, Fig. 3–13). They can then be replayed and, if desired, segments can be photographed from the oscilloscope. The magnetic tape also can be used with computers for further analysis, such as counting the number of potentials of various frequencies, amplitudes, and durations. The specifications of the tape recorder should be of sufficient quality to display the signals with minimum distortion.

A signal averager can be obtained for most commercially available ENM units. It is needed to detect weak signals which otherwise would be indistinguishable from the electronic background noise and is especially useful for detecting small sensory potentials. They also may be used to detect small signals from other slowly conducting fibers (3).

Amplifiers

Most equipment for EMG employs a "push-pull" type of electronic circuit that utilizes two recording electrodes (differential amplification). When the electrical impulses presented to these two electrodes are identical with respect to time, amplitude, frequency, and phase, only a straight-line trace is displayed on the oscilloscope. Thus only parameter differences are visualized. The advantage of this system is that, by effectively offsetting extraneous signals unavoidably present at both recording electrodes simultaneously, it provides a low noise level.

The two recording electrodes, referred to by a variety of names, both are detecting signals and are responsible for the resultant trace that is displayed. In electroencephalography, which employs similar circuitry, they are referred to as G–1 and G–2 (after the electronic grids 1 and 2 in the differential circuit). The wiring of the circuit is such that, when G–1 is negative to G–2, the response is visualized as an upgoing deflection from the baseline (in contrast to the physical sciences, physiologists designate an upgoing trace as "negative"). In ENM, G–1 is placed nearest the electrically active tissue; it is variously called the active, recording, different, or pickup electrode, while G–2 is called the indifferent or distant electrode. In this text, G–1 will be referred to as the active electrode; G–2, the indifferent electrode.

Types of Needle Electrodes

Several types of needle electrodes are available for EMG. All are constructed of conducting metals and have specific characteristics with regard to length, diameter, insulation, and impedance. They should be kept sharp at all times. Fig. 1–3A shows the types commonly employed: monopolar, concentric, coaxial (bifilar), and multielectrode.

The monopolar electrode consists of a single strand of solid, firm metal, usually steel. It is coated with Teflon along its entire length except for the distal, bared, 0.5–mm tip. A second similar electrode may be used with the monopolar electrode as the indifferent electrode. It is inserted subcutaneously within a few centimeters of the active electrode.

An indifferent surface electrode may be used instead of an indifferent needle

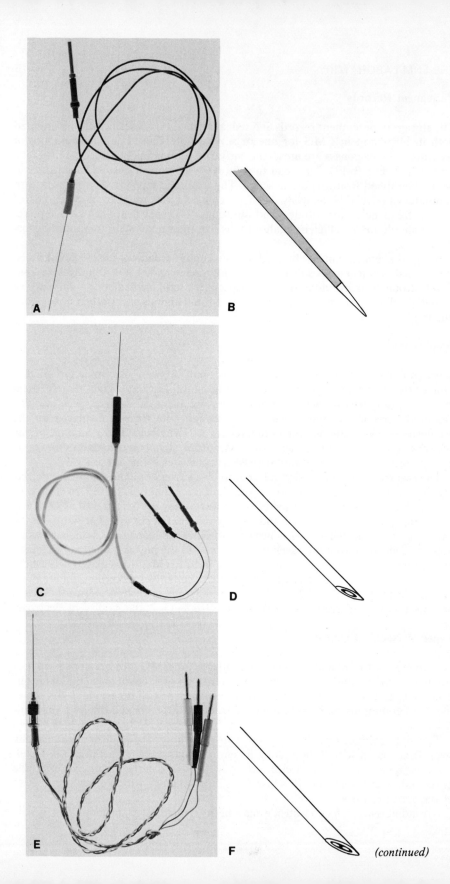

(continued)

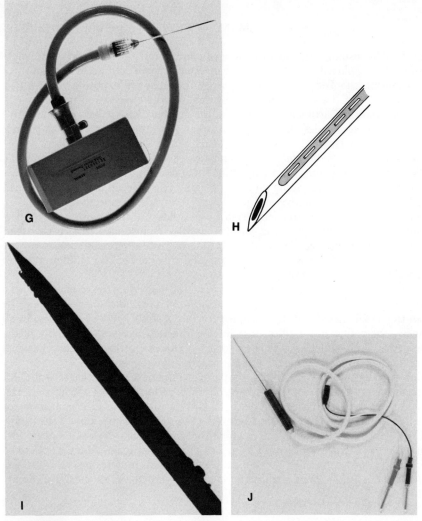

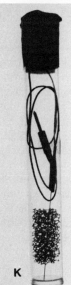

Fig. 1–3. Needle electrodes (EMG). **A-H.** Four types of needle electrodes are illustrated with a photograph of the actual needle and a diagrammatic representation of the needle tip. A and B. Monopolar. C and D. Concentric. E and F. Coaxial (bifilar). G and H. A multielectrode. **I.** A photograph of a monopolar needle with damaged Teflon coating. The coating has peeled away from the needle electrode so as to render the needle unsuitable for EMG. **J-K.** Needle electrodes packaged for sterilization. **J.** Coaxial needle electrode in plastic envelope. **K.** Needle electrode in glass tube. In either case, the needle is autoclaved and appropriately labelled as to date of sterilization.

electrode. This usually consists of a piece of conducting metal several centimeters in diameter. It is placed 2–10 cm from the inserted active electrode. With continued use (or abuse), the Teflon coating may break or wear off, exposing more of the needle (Fig. 1–3I). This will alter its electrical characteristics and produce disfigured potentials and artifacts. By virtue of the greater distance between the active and indifferent electrodes than with the other types described later, potentials appear somewhat larger.

The concentric needle electrode usually consists of a 22–gauge hypodermic needle into which a fine, solid-core wire has been inserted. This solid wire is insulated from the needle along its entire length. The wire tip and the outer shell of the needle act as the active and indifferent electrodes, respectively.

The coaxial needle electrode consists of two solid-wire cores within a hypodermic needle; each of the two wires and the needle are insulated from each other. In contrast to the concentric needle electrode, a coaxial electrode measures the difference in potential between the two exposed tips (active and indifferent) with the needle acting as the ground.

The multielectrode needle consists of a large-bore needle (16–18 gauge) with a number of insulated wires inserted with tips bared at regular intervals along the side of the needle (1). These are designed for motor–unit territory analysis. In all instances, the active and indifferent poles are attached by wire (preferably of the same electrical characteristics as the needle electrodes) to the amplifier circuit at its input. It then is circuited for visual and auditory display.

Each needle electrode is kept in a separate container, such as a test tube, for sterilization and storage. They should be checked periodically for proper electrical characteristics and sharpness. A piece of tape is placed on each container for recording the date on which it was sterilized. (Fig. 1–3K). The length of the needle used will depend on the depth the examiner needs to place it to reach and explore the muscle. Needles vary in length from 2 to 5 cm; other lengths may be obtained for special purposes. Smaller needles are used for small muscles near the surface. The concentric and monopolar needle electrodes are the ones most commonly employed.

ELECTRODIAGNOSTIC UNIT

Standard EDX equipment is designed to deliver square-wave pulses and consists of three units: 1) an amperage control and milliammeter from which the current can be read; 2) a device to control impulse duration; and 3) a provision to vary impulse interval. By means of controls, the examiner varies these parameters. Included is a control that can reverse polarity of the two electrodes. The stimulating electrode may be of various forms and sizes, but usually consists of a ball electrode covered with felt, with a spherical diameter of about one cm. The indifferent electrode is usually a wire mesh several square centimeters in area (Ch. 4, Fig. 4–3).

A number of other techniques are available in ENM which are not a part of the routine ENM procedure. These include units for *in vitro* intracellular recordings of nerve–muscle preparations (4) and single-fiber EMG; a variety of computers for assessing various parameters of potentials and EMG studies of muscle actions (kinesthesiology). The procedures for these various techniques will not be discussed in this manual.

REFERENCES

1. Buchtal F, Guld C, Rosenfalck P: Multielectrode study of the territory of a motor unit. Acta Physiol Scand [Suppl] 39: 83–104, 1957
2. Buchtal F, Rosenfalck P: Evoked action potentials and conduction velocity in human sensory nerves. Brain Res 3: 16, 1966 Special Issue
3. Buchtal F, Rosenfalck P: Sensory potentials in polyneuropathy. Brain 94: 241–262, 1971
4. Elmqvist D, Lambert EH: Detailed analysis of neuromuscular transmission in a patient with the myasthenic syndrome sometimes associated with bronchogenic carcinoma. Mayo Clin Proc 43: 689–713, 1968
5. Grass E, Grass A: Electrical Safety. Quincy, MA, Grass Instruments, 1972, p 25

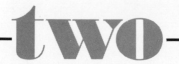

NERVE STIMULATION STUDIES

DEFINITION OF TERMS

The characteristics of neuromuscular integrity which may be ascertained by means of NSSs include: 1) the *electrical excitability* of the peripheral neuromuscular system; 2) motor and sensory *conduction latency;* 3) *conduction velocity,* both sensory and motor, of segments of the nerve; 4) the *amplitude* and *duration* of the *evoked response* (compound-muscle-action potential or nerve potential); 5) the *fatigability* of the peripheral neuromuscular system to repetitive stimulation; and 6) *reflex response* (H reflex, F wave).

In brief, the technique is as follows: Stimulating electrodes are applied to the skin surface over a nerve, or needle electrodes are placed subcutaneously adjacent to a nerve. An electric current of sufficient strength to excite the nerve then is applied. The response is detected from the "end organ," a muscle for motor studies, or, in the case of a nerve, by active and indifferent electrodes at some point along its course.

Motor conduction velocity is defined as the distance an impulse travels along a nerve per unit time. It is reported in meters per second (m/sec). Conduction velocity is not constant along the entire length of a nerve. As an impulse approaches the distal portion of a nerve where terminal branching occurs, it is slowed. There is further delay at the neuromyal junction mediated by chemical transmission. Finally an electric impulse spreads along the muscle membrane and sarcoplasmic reticulum approximately 0.5 msec prior to mechanical contraction.

In order to obtain an accurate determination of conduction velocity along the main body of the nerve, it is necessary to eliminate the time which is occupied by terminal slowing, neuromyal junction transmission, and muscle membrane events. This is accomplished by stimulating the nerve at two points separated by a reasonable distance but proximal to terminal branching. Thus two responses are obtained utilizing the same muscle for the evoked response. The time from the onset of the applied electric stimulus to the onset of the response of the more distal stimulation

10

site is subtracted from the analogous value from the more proximal site (Fig. 2–1). The distance between the stimulation sites then is divided by the value which results from subtracting the distal from the proximal time (the time for the impulse to travel this segment). The result is the motor NCV for that segment of nerve. Any alteration or abnormality in NCV refers to that portion of the nerve which has been measured.

The time from onset of stimulus to onset of response is termed *motor latency time* or more briefly *latency*. *Latency rate* may be calculated when only one point along the nerve is stimulated. It is defined as the distance from a single point of stimulation to the site of response divided by the time taken by the impulse to traverse this distance. This value includes the transmission events at the distal end of the nerve. It may be compared with other homologous latencies, but not with the NCV.

In contrast to motor stimulation studies, *sensory stimulation studies* do not have the added variable of neuromyal junction delay. The results may be recorded as *latency* in milliseconds (msec) at a stipulated distance or as *velocity* in meters per second (m/sec). Several recording sites may be used to determine the velocity along various segments of the nerve.

Repetitive stimulation consists of repeated electrical stimuli at specific rates

Fig. 2–1. Principles of motor nerve conduction. The figure illustrates the positions of stimulating and recording electrodes for median nerve motor conduction study. **1.** Stimulating electrodes over nerve, proximal position. **2.** Stimulating electrodes over nerve, distal position. **3.** Position of the recording electrodes, the active electrode over the thenar eminence and the indifferent electrode on the thumb. The ground is illustrated in the palm. **1–3.** Resultant trace when nerve is stimulated at *1*. First vertical deflection, stimulus artifact; second vertical deflection, onset of compound-muscle-action potential. **2–3.** As in *1-3* above, but from distal stimulation site. In each case, the time from the first to the second vertical deflection is the respective latency.

$$\text{LR (latency rate)} = \frac{\text{distance } (d) \text{ } 1\text{–}3}{\text{latency } (t) \text{ } 1\text{–}3}$$

or on distal stimulation

$$\text{LR} = \frac{(d) \text{ } 2\text{–}3}{(t) \text{ } 2\text{–}3}$$

$$\text{Nerve conduction velocity (NCV)} = \frac{\text{distance } (d) \text{ } 1\text{–}2}{[\text{latency } (t) \text{ } 1\text{–}3] - [\text{latency } (t) \text{ } 2\text{–}3]}$$

Where t = time in msec, d = distance in mm, and NCV is measured in meters per second.

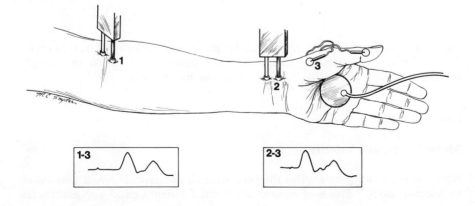

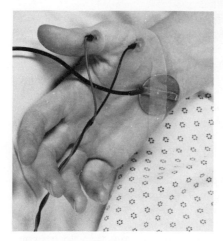

Fig. 2–2. Surface and ground electrodes secured with highly adhesive translucent tape.

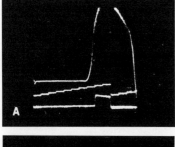

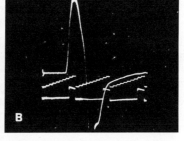

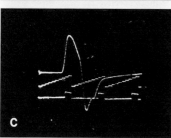

Fig. 2–3. Compound-muscle-action potential, effect of proper and improper gain and sweep speed. Stimulation of median nerve at elbow. In each set: top trace, response to stimulation; center trace, time, 1 msec/step; bottom trace, calibration, 1 mV. **A.** Amplitude and duration of trace incompletely shown. **B.** Vertical position of potential off screen (clipping). **C.** Potential completely recorded.

applied to a nerve at one site and recorded from a muscle innervated by that nerve. This technique evaluates the integrity of the neuromyal junction to multiple stimuli, especially electrochemical events across the synapse.

PROCEDURE

Motor Conduction Velocity

Before the test is begun, explain the procedure to the patient. Avoid terms such as "electric shock." This is often associated in the patient's mind with electrocon-

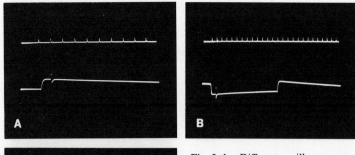

Fig. 2–4. Different oscilloscope sweep speeds and their effect on calibration signal wave form. **A, B** and *C* represent the same calibration signal (bottom line of each trace) photographed at three different sweep speeds. In each trace the top line is a 1 msec time base. The sweep speed becomes progressively slower *A* to *C*.

Fig. 2–5. Measurement of NCV, and amplitude and duration of the compound-muscle-action potentials. **A.** Stimulation of median nerve at elbow. Upper trace-*arrow* at onset of compound-muscle-action potential. Middle trace—one msec per step. Bottom trace—Calibration, one mV. **B.** As above, stimulation at wrist. **C.** Median nerve sensory action potential, recorded at the index finger with stimulation at the wrist. Calibration, 100 μV. Measured Values: In *A,* motor latency, 8.4 msec; amplitude, action potential, 10 mV; duration, action potential, 10.6 msec. In *B,* motor latency, 3.2 msec; amplitude, action potential, 10.5 mV; duration, action potential, 11.3 msec. Distance between two points of stimulation (elbow to wrist), 250 mm.In *C*, latency, 2.3 msec; amplitude, 18 μV; duration, 2.7 msec. Calculated values:

$$\text{NCV} = \frac{d}{t} = \frac{250}{(8.4 - 3.2)} = \frac{250}{5.2} = 48.1 \text{ m/sec.}$$

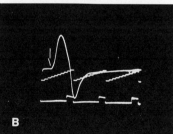

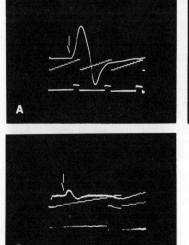

vulsive therapy or some regrettable experience with electricity. One should emphasize that it is a test and not a treatment, and that, during one portion of the test,
electrical impulses are "fed" into different nerves to see how well they are working.
The patient must be relaxed, and it is especially important that the muscles of the
extremity be at rest.

The skin over those areas where the stimulating and recording electrodes are to
be applied should be cleansed with alcohol. This will remove extraneous dirt and
oil from the skin, allowing better contact of electrodes with the skin surface and
reduction of resistance. Under certain circumstances, e.g., when testing an edematous limb, needle electrodes may be used instead of the customary surface type both
to record and stimulate in order to obtain a measurable response with the least
current. The patient should be instructed to tell the examiner if a particularly
painful area is being probed so that the needle may be moved. The routine use of
needle electrodes for NCV studies has the disadvantage of additional discomfort
and the need for sterile equipment, but usually less current is used for supramaximal stimulation and the time values are shortened by as much as 1.0 msec. This
may produce a difference of up to 10 m/sec in some conduction velocities (44).

All surface electrodes—stimulating, recording, and ground—should be moistened with electrode paste before being placed on the skin (this does not apply to
needle electrodes). In motor NSS, the active electrode is placed over the belly of
the muscle as close to the endplate zone as possible. If this electrode is not placed
properly over the endplate region, the contour of the action potential will be
changed and error introduced (5). The indifferent electrode is placed 3–4 cm
distal to, but not over, the muscle (group) being tested (whenever possible), usually over the tendon of the muscle or a bony prominence close by. The electrodes
are secured to the skin with tape (Fig. 2–2). Nonallergic, highly adhesive, translucent skin tape is available commercially. The ground electrode usually is placed
between the point of stimulation and the recording electrode. This serves to reduce the shock artifact.

After the recording and ground electrodes are in place and before stimulation
of the nerve, the equipment should be checked carefully to insure proper settings
of the following: 1) electrode placement; 2) stimulation sites; 3) stimulus intensity
settings: duration of impulse, voltage or amperage; 4) oscilloscope adjustments:
focus, intensity of trace, vertical position of trace, sweep speed; and 5) calibration
and time–base marker (which should be included with each record). The sweep
speed of the oscilloscope should be changed according to the situation so that the
entire electrical event can be recorded and analyzed (Figs. 2–3 and 2–4, and
Summary of Steps in performing NSS, Step 10).

In practice, the motor conduction velocity of a peripheral nerve is obtained by
placing the stimulating electrode on the skin directly over the nerve. Palpation of
the nerve bundle, when possible, is a valuable guide to placement of the electrodes.
If the stimulating cathode is not close to the nerve, a false increase in latency will
occur. Start with a very low voltage to allow the patient to become familiar with
the sensation of the impulse. The voltage then is increased rapidly until just
supramaximal response is obtained, delivering a single stimulus at each voltage
increment. Supramaximal response has been reached when no further increase in
the amplitude of the action potential is apparent with a slight increase in stimulus
voltage. When this response has been obtained, it is recorded.

The procedure is repeated at another point along the nerve as far from the first
stimulation point as reasonable. The actual distance between the two points of
stimulation is then measured (in millimeters) along the extremity with a tape

measure. This distance should reflect the course of the nerve as closely as possible. The time taken for the impulse to travel between these two points is used to calculate the conduction velocity of the nerve (Fig. 2–5).

$$\text{NCV} = \frac{\text{distance }(d)}{\text{time }(t)} = \frac{\text{millimeters}}{\text{millisecond}} = \frac{\text{meters}}{\text{second}}$$

In some instances when a second point of stimulation is difficult or even impossible to obtain, the latency time is ascertained even though NCV more accurately reflects impulse travel along the nerve segment.

The principle of motor NCV can be applied to several segments of a nerve. For example, the ulnar nerve can be stimulated below the elbow using the compound-muscle-action potential of the hypothenar muscles as the endpoint for recording. With the same endpoint, the ulnar nerve can be stimulated at the midarm, axilla, and wrist. Conduction velocity of each segment may be calculated by subtraction of successively distal segments. In this way, significant slowing from compression of the nerve about the elbow can be detected and differentiated from lesions elsewhere.

The amplitude of compound muscle action potentials is measured in millivolts; duration, in milliseconds. The amplitude is measured in centimeters from the baseline to the point of maximum negative deflection of the trace. This distance is converted to millivolts by comparing it with the known deflection of the calibration signal (Fig. 2–5). Thus, if the calibration signal deflection is 2.0 cm for 1 mV and the compound-muscle-action potential is 1.5 cm, the amplitude is $\frac{1.5}{2.0} \times 1 = 0.75$ mV. Duration of the response can be measured in several ways. One common method is to measure the distance from the onset of the response to the point at which the trace first crosses the baseline. This measures the negative phase of the response. One also can measure from the onset of the potential to the point at which the trace returns to the baseline, but this is sometimes difficult to determine in actual practice, especially if the response is abnormal.

The area subtended under the curve can be measured with a planimeter or electronically. This technique can be used, for example, in instances when a patient is being tested periodically to note the return of function (13).

Fig. 2–6. Sensory action potential with and without averaging technique. Stimulation of the median nerve at the wrist and recording from the index finger in a patient with carpal tunnel syndrome. **A.** Top trace, single stimulus. Note that no potential can be detected from the background noise. Center trace, time base (1 msec/step). Bottom trace, averaged response (about 50 sweeps). Sensory latency, 4.3 msec to onset of response and 5.2 msec to peak. **B.** Calibration for A = 10 μV.

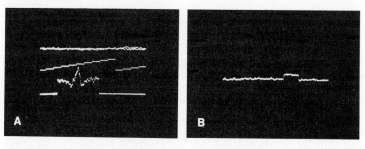

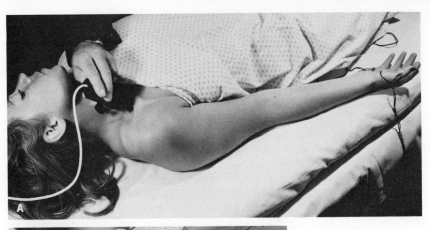

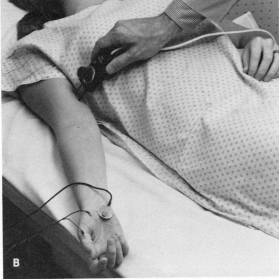

(continued)

Fig. 2–7. Motor NCV study, median nerve. **A.** Stimulation at Erb's point with recording electrode over the thenar eminence. **B.** Stimulation at mid arm level. **C.** Stimulation at anticubital fossa. **D.** Stimulation at wrist.

Sensory Conduction Studies

Measurements of *sensory conduction* differ from measurements of motor conduction in that terminal slowing is not a significant factor. Sensory conduction may be measured from a distal site of stimulation (e.g., a finger) to the onset of the evoked response along the nerve bundle. This is recorded from electrodes placed in proximal position over the corresponding nerve. Before the availability of equipment with a high signal-to-noise ratio and averaging techniques, it was more convenient to measure the peak of the nerve-action potential. In most instances, modern equipment permits measurement to the onset of the response. Responses

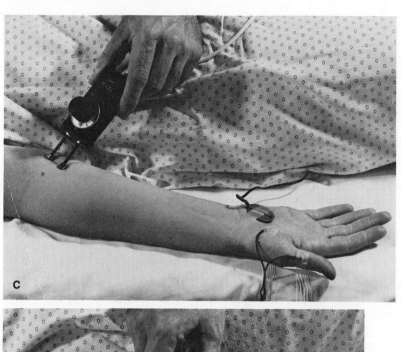

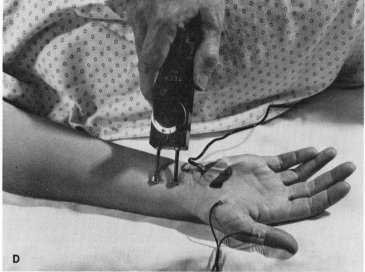

are reported as sensory conduction latency (milliseconds) or velocity (meters per second) (Fig. 2–6).

SPECIFIC STIMULATION STUDIES

Nerve stimulation studies received their greatest impetus from the work of Erlanger and Gasser (1925–1929) (12) and Hodes, Larabee, and German (18). At present, with adequate equipment, most peripheral nerves can be assessed electrically.

The examiner may change the sites of stimulation and recording from those suggested later to adjust to a particular clinical situation. When needle electrodes are used for stimulation and recording, nerves—especially sensory branches—not readily accessible by surface stimulation become available.

Individual peripheral nerves will be considered separately.

Motor Nerve Stimulation Studies

When the *median nerve* is to be stimulated for motor studies, place the active electrode at the center of the thenar eminence, and the indifferent electrode at the base of the first phalanx of the thumb. The ground electrode usually is placed on the palmar or dorsal surface of the hand. If the shock artifact appears too large, the ground can be moved to another site between the stimulating and recording electrodes.

The median nerve can be stimulated at various sites: wrist, elbow, midarm, axilla, and brachial plexus. The cathode of the stimulator initiates the stimulus. Therefore it always is placed in apposition to (closest to) the active recording electrode to produce the shortest latency. Failure to do this prolongs the latency (Fig. 2–21D).

To stimulate the nerve at the wrist, the cathode is placed between the tendons of the palmaris longus and the flexor carpi radialis muscles, just proximal to the transverse carpal ligament. The anode is in a proximal position relative to the cathode (avoid simultaneous stimulation of the ulnar nerve) (Fig. 2–7D). To stimulate the median nerve at the level of the elbow, the cathode is placed just medial to the brachial artery at about the center of the cubital fossa with the anode in proximal position (Fig. 2–7C).

More proximal lesions of the median nerve can be studied by stimulation at the level of the midarm and supraclavicular fossa (Figs. 2–7A and B). The nerve lies in proximity to the brachial artery along the medial aspect of the arm. The NCV of each segment can be estimated by measuring the appropriate distances and latencies. For example, if the latency from the midarm is 9 msec and from the elbow is 7 msec, then the time from midarm to elbow is $9 - 7 = 2$ msec. If the corresponding distance is 110 cm, then the NCV for this segment is $\frac{110}{2.0} = 55$ m/sec. Very short distances, less than 10 cm, may introduce error in the NCV value because of the difficulty involved in accurate measurement of short segments.

For an *ulnar nerve* study, the active electrode is placed midway along the lateral border of the hypothenar eminence, and the indifferent electrode is placed at the base of the proximal phalanx of the fifth finger. When the deep perforating branch of the ulnar nerve is to be tested, place the active electrode over the first dorsal interosseous muscle with the indifferent electrode just distal to the base of the second phalanx of the thumb. The ground electrode should be placed as described earlier.

At the wrist, the cathode is placed just medial to the tendon of the flexor carpi ulnaris muscle at about the same level as indicated for the median nerve (Fig. 2–8A). Here the anode should be placed on the ulnar side of the nerve to avoid simultaneous stimulation of the median nerve. For stimulation at the elbow, the stimulating electrode is placed in the ulnar notch in the vicinity of the medial epicondyle (Fig. 2–8B). When a lesion at the elbow is suspected, stimulate several centimeters proximal and distal to the elbow as described above for the median nerve.

When clinical indications require, the ulnar nerve can be stimulated in other locations, including the axilla and along the groove between the biceps and triceps muscles on the medial surface of the forearm over the neurovascular bundle (Fig. 2–8C) and at the brachial plexus at Erb's point (Fig. 2–7A). These do not necessarily form part of every NCV study.

To stimulate the *radial nerve,* place the cathode of the stimulator along the posterolateral aspect of the arm between the brachialis and triceps muscles (Fig. 2–9A). The second site of stimulation may be at the cubital fossa just medial to the brachioradialis muscle (Fig. 2–9B). The active electrode is placed over the center of the extensor digitorum communis muscle and the indifferent electrode distal to it.

The radial nerve can also be stimulated at Erb's point or in the axilla just behind the anterior axillary fold, with the recording electrode over the belly of the triceps muscle and the reference electrode over the tendon (Fig. 2–13). The ground electrode is placed between the stimulating and recording electrodes (15).

The response of the *peroneal nerve* generally is recorded from the extensor digitorum brevis muscle. The active electrode is placed over the most prominent portion of the muscle and the indifferent electrode distally near the outer edge of the foot. The ground electrode should be placed over the dorsum of the foot or the ankle. To stimulate the peroneal nerve at the knee, the cathode usually is placed inside the lateral border of the popliteal fossa medial to the head of the fibula (Fig. 2–10A). The position of the anode, as noted above, should be proximal to the cathode.

Stimulation of the peroneal nerve at the ankle may be difficult at times, especially if the leg is edematous. The terminal branches of the nerve usually are located just lateral to the tendon of the long toe extensors, slightly below the level of the ankle (lateral malleolus) (Fig. 2–10B).

When clinical indications arise, such as in patients with crossed-leg palsy, the peroneal nerve can be stimulated at a third point just distal and anterior to the head of the fibula. This technique will demonstrate the point at which the nerve has been injured, because stimulation of the nerve in the popliteal fossa will evoke no response (or a small compound muscle action potential), whereas stimulation at the second site below the point of injury will do so. An analogous technique is used at the elbow in the ulnar groove in cases of tardy ulnar palsy.

For stimulation of the *posterior tibial nerve,* the cathode of the stimulator is placed in the central portion of the popliteal space with the anode proximal in position (Fig. 2–11A). The active electrode is placed over the belly of one of the plantar muscles on the plantar surface of the foot, with the reference electrode on the lateral aspect of the fifth toe. With the electrode in this position, the tibial nerve is stimulated at a second point at the ankle just behind the medial malleolus (Fig. 2–11B).

The *sciatic nerve* can be stimulated by placing the cathode on the buttock either between the greater trochanter of the femur and the tuberosity of the ischium or directly below the middle of this position on a line drawn downward to the apex of the popliteal fossa (16, 44). A needle electrode inserted near the nerve may be required for stimulation. The second point of stimulation is the posterior tibial nerve, posterior to the middle portion of the medial malleolus, in a manner analo-

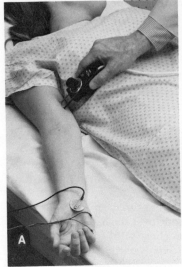

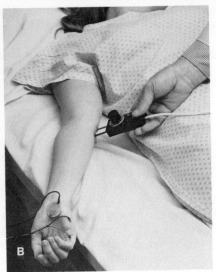

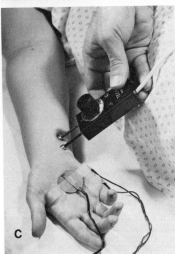

Fig. 2–8.   Motor NCV, ulnar nerve. **A.** Stimulation at midarm. **B.** Stimulation at elbow. **C.** Stimulation at wrist. Stimulation at Erb's point is identical with Fig. 2–7A except that the recording electrodes are over the hypothenar eminence.

gous to that already described. In this way, the conduction velocity along the entire sciatic nerve is measured, including the posterior tibial nerve. The response of the latter, as well as that of the sciatic nerve, should be recorded from the plantar muscles (44).

Latency Studies

When a second point of stimulation along a peripheral nerve is not feasible, latency, rather than NCV, is measured. The recording electrode is placed a predetermined distance from the point of stimulation. The values obtained from an individual patient then are compared with the normal range for that nerve at that specified

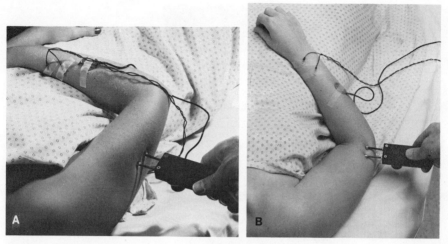

Fig. 2–9. Motor NCV radial nerve. **A.** Proximal point of stimulation with recording electrode over the extensor digitorum communis. **B.** Distal point of stimulation, otherwise same as *A*.

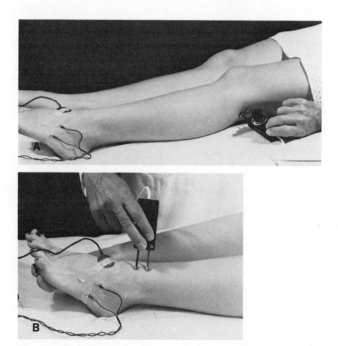

Fig. 2–10. Motor NCV peroneal nerve. **A.** Proximal point of stimulation and proximal to the head of the fibula. Recording electrode over the extensor digitorum brevis. **B.** Distal point of stimulation.

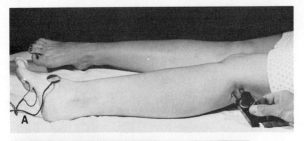

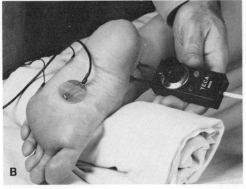

Fig. 2–11. Motor NCV posterior tibial nerve. **A.** Proximal point of stimulation in the popliteal fossa. **B.** Distal point of stimulation just inferior to the medial malleolus. For purposes of illustration, the patient is prone in this second figure. This study can be done in the supine position with equal ease. In this study, the recording electrode is on at the abductor digiti V. At the examiner's discretion, the pickup electrode may be placed over the abductor hallucis muscle near the head of the first metatarsal bone on the plantar surface of the foot.

Fig. 2–12. Latency, facial nerve. Stimulation of the facial nerve above the angle of the jaw. Recording electrode over the orbicularis oris, 10 cm from the stimulating electrode. Indifferent electrode over the chin.

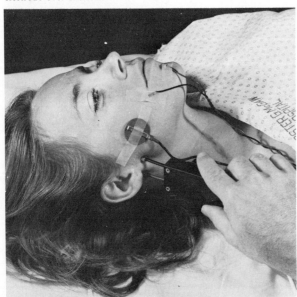

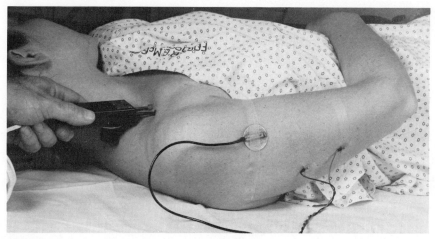

Fig. 2–13. Latency, radial nerve. Stimulation at Erb's point with recording electrodes over the triceps muscle 25 cm distal to the cathode.

distance. The facial, musculocutaneous and femoral nerves are among those that lend themselves better to latency than to NCV studies.

The *facial nerve* is stimulated just before it enters the parotid gland anterior to the lobe of the ear (Fig. 2–12). One of several muscles may be selected for recording; for example, above the eyebrow (frontalis), at the outer canthus of the eye (orbicularis oculi), or near the corner of the mouth (orbicularis oris). The site of recording is dictated by the nature of the problem and the clinical examination; when one or two branches of the nerve have been traumatized, the appropriate muscle should be chosen for recording.

The indifferent electrode is placed several centimeters distally from the active electrode; the bridge of the nose or the midline of the forehead or chin are good sites for the indifferent electrode. The ground electrode is placed between the stimulating and recording electrodes. The result obtained by this procedure is a latency, because the nerve is stimulated at only one point along its course. The latency rate may be calculated by dividing the distance between the stimulating and recording electrodes by the time from the stimulus artifact to the beginning of the action potential. Always compare the clinically involved side with the normal side (25).

For study of the *femoral nerve,* the stimulating electrodes are placed along the course of the nerve as it emerges beneath the inguinal ligament and courses down the anterior surface of the thigh (Fig. 2–14). The recording electrodes are placed over the belly of the vastus intermedius muscle at a measured distance away (14–16 cm), with the indifferent electrode in distal position.

Latency time for the deltoid, biceps, supraspinatus, and infraspinatus muscles can be obtained by stimulating the brachial plexus in the supraclavicular fossa and recording from appropriate sites (Fig. 2–15) (9, 15). In lesions of the brachial plexus, this technique is quite valuable. A prolonged latency may reflect pathology in discrete parts of the plexus as well as in the main body.

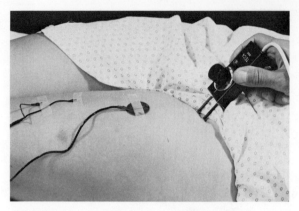

Fig. 2–14. Latency, femoral nerve. Recording electrode over the vastus intermedius 16 cm distal to the stimulating electrode over the femoral nerve. Electrodes, from right to left: stimulating, ground, active, and indifferent.

Fig. 2–15. Brachial plexus latencies. **A.** To deltoid muscle (axillary nerve). Recording electrode over the deltoid muscle, 15 cm distal to the stimulating electrode over Erb's point. **B.** To biceps brachii (musculocutaneous nerve). Recording electrode over the biceps brachii, 24 cm distal to the stimulating electrode over Erb's point.

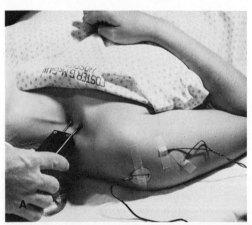

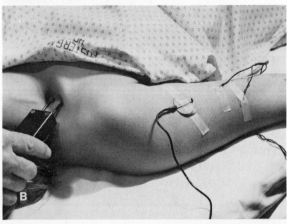

Sensory Nerve Stimulation Studies

The amplitude of sensory responses from nerves are much smaller than the compound-muscle-action potentials discussed above and may be difficult to distinguish from the background noise. Several methods are used to overcome this difficulty: 1) needle (rather than surface) electrodes for recording can be placed in proximity to the nerve; 2) multiple responses can be superimposed on the oscilloscope screen to help distinguish background noise from the action potential; and, 3) most effectively, a signal averager may be used. The last technique has the advantage of showing weak signals clearly because random background activity is reduced significantly. However, nonrandom responses also will be additive; e.g., artifacts, cross-talk pulse and muscle responses.

As with motor NCV studies, the responses from the fastest fibers are measured (techniques have been described to detect the responses of the slower conducting sensory fibers) (4).

It always is best to perform motor NCV studies first to find the exact location of the nerve and any anatomic variations. These loci are marked on the skin so that the recording electrodes can be placed at the identical sites.

METHOD I: ORTHODROMIC   Sensory conduction velocity for the *median* and *ulnar nerves* is measured with the stimulating electrodes placed over the index and fifth fingers, respectively, and the recording electrodes at the wrist (Fig. 2–16A) or in one of several more proximal positions. Several types of stimulating electrodes are available: 1) expandable ring electrodes; 2) "alligator clamp" electrodes; 3) pipe cleaners soaked in saline; 4) the same electrodes used for motor nerve stimulation; and 5) needle electrodes in proximity to a nerve. The choice depends upon the nerve to be stimulated and its location.

Using the median nerve as an example, the cathode is placed at the base of the index finger and the anode is placed 2–3 cm distal to this point. The active electrode is positioned over the median nerve at the wrist at the same point where the stimulating cathode was placed for motor NCV study. The indifferent electrode is placed in a proximal position 2–3 cm away. It is important to have a secure ground electrode when performing these studies. The amplifier sensitivity should be set at a higher gain (usually between 10 and 100 μV). Ulnar nerve sensory conduction is determined in an analogous manner; radial nerve sensory conduction measurements also have been described (9).

One also may place the recording electrodes over the median and ulnar nerves at the elbow (or even more proximally) and perform the test in a similar fashion. If these nerves are stimulated at the wrist and the response is recorded at the elbow, one must bear in mind that antidromic stimulation of the motor nerve may be responsible for the nerve action potential.

METHOD II: ANTIDROMIC   An alternative method for determining sensory conduction velocity employs the principle of antidromic conduction along a nerve (32). In contrast to the orthodromic method where only the sensory nerves of the fingers are stimulated, a mixed (motor and sensory) nerve is stimulated and recording is from the sensory fibers in the fingers. This method has the advantage of producing a larger nerve action potential. The procedure is the same as that described above for motor NCV studies, except that the recording electrodes are placed on the

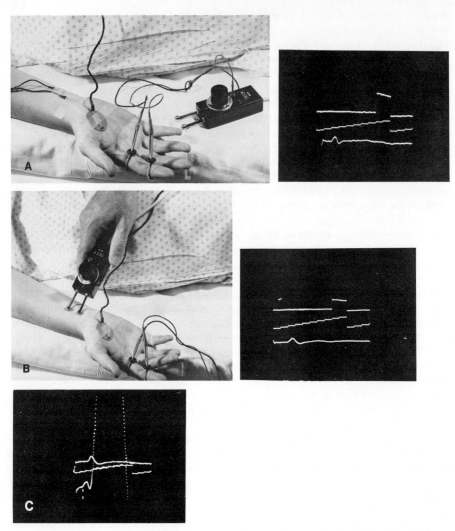

Fig. 2–16.   Sensory latency, median nerve. **A.** Method I, orthodromic. Stimulating electrodes on finger, cathode proximal to anode, 13 cm from recording electrode over median nerve at wrist. Latency = 2.0 msec. Calibration, 100 μV. Temperature = 36.8°C. **B.** Method II, antidromic. Recording electrodes on finger, recording proximal to indifferent, 13 cm distal to stimulating electrode over median nerve at wrist. Latency = 2.0 msec. Calibration, 100 μV. **C.** Simultaneous display of sensory (top trace) and motor (bottom trace) responses from median nerve. The crest of the compound-muscle-action potential is off the screen due to the gain required to detect the sensory potential. The onset of the nerve action potential ("n" potential) is seen just prior to the muscle action potential (vertical dashes). Calibration, as in *B*. Sensory latency = 2.5 msec; motor latency 3.0 msec.

proximal (active) and distal (indifferent) phalanges of the appropriate finger, and the stimulating electrodes are over the nerve at the wrist (Fig. 2–16B).

Sensory stimulation of the upper extremity sometimes affords a method of distinguishing nerve root from brachial plexus lesions. When the nerves have been interrupted at the level of the brachial plexus, there is degeneration of the sensory as well as the motor fibers. With a lesion of the nerve roots proximal to the sensory neuron cell body in the dorsal root ganglion, the distal sensory nerve fiber does not degenerate (although sensation is lost as a result of interruption of the proximal branch to the spinal cord).

Stimulation of the sensory nerves of the fingers with proximal recording of the appropriate nerve can detect the responses for C-6 (thumb-index fingers), C-7 (index-middle fingers), and C-8 (ring-fifth fingers). Thus, for example, with a brachial plexus lesion involving the C-7 fibers, stimulation of the middle finger (recording from the median nerve at the wrist or elbow) will evoke no response; if the lesion is at the root level with the sensory neuron cell body intact, a response will be obtained (this presupposes that degeneration already has taken place).

Antidromic stimulation of the *sural nerve* is accomplished by placing the active electrodes posterior to the lateral aspect of the ankle near its inferior border where there is usually a slight depression. The indifferent electrode is placed 3–4 cm distal to it. The sural nerve is stimulated at several sites proximal to the active electrode. The nerve can be stimulated, for example, at 7, 14, and 21 cm from the active electrode (Fig. 2–17A). A signal averager is especially useful when stimulating diseased nerve because the nerve action potential is very small. Sensory stimulation studies of other nerves, e.g., axillary, peroneal (Fig. 2–17B), and radial have been reported (3, 6, 26).

H REFLEX AND F WAVE

The H reflex is a stimulus–response described in 1920 by Hoffman (19, 20). It was investigated further in 1950 by Magladery and McDougal (27). The impulse produced by submaximal stimulation of a peripheral nerve travels the sensory fibers to the spinal cord where there is a synapse with the alpha motor neurons. An efferent impulse is initiated (after synaptic transmission) and is conducted via the motor fibers to the muscle where the compound-muscle-action potential is detected. Thus, afferent and efferent nerve fibers are involved together with a synapse in the gray matter of the spinal cord. Submaximal stimuli just over threshold excite the IA afferent fibers before the efferent, since the latter have a higher threshold. The IA afferents travel the dorsal root and then synapse in the spinal cord with the IA alpha efferent fibers. The latter conduct the impulse to the muscle and produce the H reflex, with a latency of 30–50 msec because of the distance travelled. As the stimulus intensity is increased, the efferent fibers going directly to the muscle reach threshold and the evoked response is elicited (M or direct response). But the motor fibers also conduct antidromically to the spinal cord, where they meet the orthodromic impulses described above and occlude. Thus, as the M response grows in amplitude with increased stimulus strength, the H reflex wanes: It no longer is detectable with supramaximal stimulation.

Suprasegmental control influences and modifies the H reflex. In normal individuals, the H-reflex is most readily elicited from the posterior tibial nerve, recording from the gastrocnemius muscle. Its amplitude increases in diseases of the upper

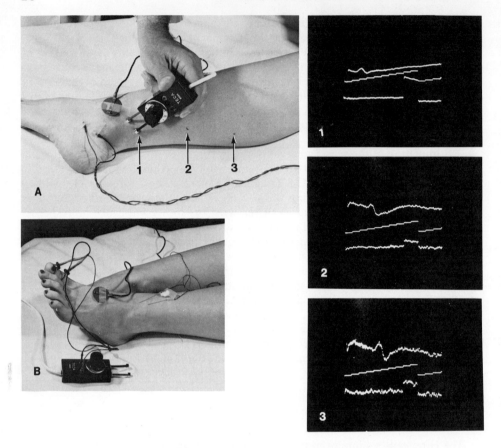

Fig. 2–17. Sensory latencies, sural and peroneal nerves. **A.** Sensory latency, sural nerve (antidromic). Surface electrodes over sural nerve at ankle; stimulating electrode (cathode) over sural nerve. The most distal of the three points of stimulation is illustrated; the two more proximal points are indicated by *arrows*. These points are respectively 7, 14, and 21 cm proximal to the recording electrode. All three responses are illustrated. The latencies, top to bottom, are: 7 cm, 1.8 msec; 14 cm, 3.2 msec; 21 cm, 4.2 msec. Calibration: 100, 10, and 10 μV, respectively. **B.** Sensory latency, peroneal nerve (averaged response, antidromic). Needle electrodes adjacent to peroneal nerve; stimulating electrodes over hallux, cathode proximal to anode.

motor neuron; it then can be obtained from the ulnar, median, and radial nerves. It also is augmented in disorders of the extrapyramidal system. In infants, the H reflex normally is present in many nerves. In lesions of the peripheral nerve, the H reflex usually is abolished. It also may be used to evaluate impairment of the sensory portion of the nerve in the absence of any motor deficit (42).

The stimulating and recording electrodes should be arranged as described for motor NCV studies of the posterior tibial nerve. The strength of the stimulus gradually is increased, beginning with a minimal amount. On the oscilloscope, at about 30–35 msec from the stimulus artifact, a small action potential will be seen. This is the H reflex (Fig. 2–18). A minimal increase in the strength of the stimulus

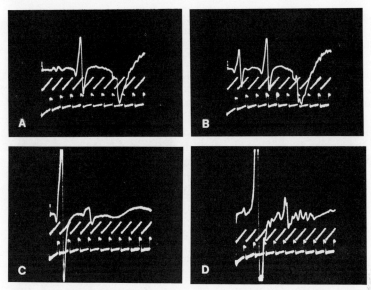

Fig. 2–18. H reflex, M response, and F wave. Recording from the left gastrocnemius with surface electrodes, stimulating the posterior tibial nerve in the popliteal fossa. Calibration, 100 μV; 10 msec/staircase. **A.** Minimal stimulus: H reflex appears at 32 msec. **B.** Submaximal stimulus: H reflex persists and M response begins to appear at 6 msec. **C.** Submaximal stimulus greater than B: H reflex almost gone and M response more fully developed at 6 msec. **D.** Supramaximal stimulus: F wave appears at 44 msec.

Fig. 2–19. Repetitive stimulation, median nerve. Recording electrode over thenar eminence, stimulating electrodes over median nerve. The arm and hand have been fixed firmly to a moulded support by Velcro straps (other similar devices can be used).

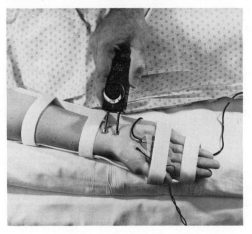

enlarges this action potential. Now a direct response also is seen but at a much shorter latency than the onset of the H reflex. Subsequently, the first response (H reflex) begins to diminish until, with supramaximal stimulation, it disappears entirely.

Another response, called the F wave (Fig. 2–18), was noted by Magladery and McDougal (27). This compound-muscle-action potential occurs near the region of the H reflex but is of somewhat longer latency. It occurs after the H reflex is abolished and the M wave is well developed. The nature of the F wave was elucidated further by Dawson and Merton (7) and Thorne (41). Strong stimulation produces not only an orthodromic impulse directly to the muscle (M response), but also an antidromic motor nerve impulse to the motor neuron pool within the anterior gray matter of the spinal cord. This initiates another response from the anterior horn cells. Although it rarely is used clinically, it can be employed to test the excitability of the more proximal portion of the motor nerve in some clinical situations (22).

NEUROMYAL JUNCTION STUDIES

The presence of neuromyal junction dysfunction can be demonstrated by repetitive stimulation studies. Two indications for such studies are myasthenia gravis and the myasthenic syndrome of Lambert-Eaton (24). Other disorders of the neuromuscular apparatus may have a small conduction defect as a component of the disease, e.g., amyotrophic lateral sclerosis and polymyositis. The electroneuromyographer should be alerted to the presence of such a disorder when the amplitude of the compound-muscle-action potential appears to decrease during NCV studies. In myasthenia gravis, only certain muscle groups may be involved clinically; these are the ones which should be examined because an uninvolved area may not show the defect. Newer techniques to detect junctional defects have been developed (10, 11, 36).

Although repetitive stimulation studies employ some of the same procedural techniques as NCV studies, additional physiological mechanisms (inhibition, facilitation, refractory period, etc.) may become operative once multiple stimuli are delivered to the neuromyal apparatus. The extremity which is tested should be secured firmly to a mechanical device to 1) maintain a constant stretch on the muscle and 2) keep the recording electrodes in the same position (Fig. 2–19). The stimulating electrodes likewise should be held securely in the same position throughout the study. Supramaximal stimuli must be used because submaximal stimulation can produce a false–positive decrement in the amplitude of the response in normal individuals.

Several different frequencies of stimulation should be employed in these studies. In general, the normal myoneural junction will not show fatigue with stimuli under 20/sec for periods of 10–30 sec. The use of high-frequency stimulation, above 30/sec, may lead to false–positive results in normal individuals. Repetitive stimulation is painful and trains of stimuli longer than 10–20 sec should not be used under ordinary circumstances.

Fatigability of the neuromuscular unit is reflected by a decline in the amplitude of the compound-muscle-action potential to repetitive supramaximal stimulation. Using the techniques described, a consistent, reproducible progressive falloff of 25% or greater is significant. Stimulation of several muscles can increase positive findings in myasthenia gravis considerably (31).

In practice, a distal point on a nerve, such as median or ulnar at the wrist, is stimulated for several seconds at 3, 5, 10, and 20 stimuli/sec. If no defect is detected, the procedure should be repeated after vigorous exercise of the muscle for 2 min. In myasthenia gravis, the usual response is a progressive decrement of the compound-muscle-action potential (Fig. 2–20). In some rare instances, an incrementing response can be seen in patients with myasthenia gravis (34). In the myasthenic syndrome, stimulation should be preceeded by a period of rest. Supramaximal stimuli then will show an initial small response followed by a progressive increase in amplitude (and then, on some occasions, a decline). In this condition, no alteration of the response to repetitive stimulation may be noted immediately after vigorous exercise. Techniques using paired stimuli while time interval between them is varied also have been described (21).

Figure 2–20 shows two acceptable methods of display. Measurements of the response are made directly from such records to quantify the nature and degree of defect (the percentage of decrement or facilitation should be reported, together with the frequency of stimulation).

Edrophonium (Tensilon) Test

In patients with myasthenia gravis, the diagnosis can be documented by repetitive stimulation studies performed before and after administration of anticholinesterase medication. This technique also may help to differentiate between the neuromuscular fatigue of myasthenia gravis which usually responds to anticholinesterase medication and that found in the myasthenic syndrome which does not. This is accomplished by the intravenous injection of 10 mg edrophonium.

This drug must be used with due respect for its side effects: sweating, cramps, and muscle fasciculations. A test dose of 2 mg (0.2 ml) is given first because severe bradycardia or even cardiac arrest may develop if the entire dose of 10 mg (1 ml) is given rapidly at one time. In practice, three injections are given: first 0.2 ml (2 mg); then 0.3 ml (3 mg) 60 sec later; and, finally, 0.5 ml (5 mg) 2 min after the first injection. The effects of edrophonium usually subsides within 15 min. If signs of overdosage occur after the first 0.2-ml injection, the remainder is not given.

Side effects, especially bradycardia, can be counteracted by atropine, 0.4 mg IV. It is important to have a syringe of atropine filled and ready at all times. The test should be performed with at least two trained persons present in case of respiratory or cardiac arrest from overdosage. Atropine will counteract all side effects except respiratory arrest which is a skeletal muscle effect. Repetitive stimulation is applied 1 min after the last injection to demonstrate reversal of the amplitude decrement of the compound-muscle-action potential.

PATHOPHYSIOLOGY OF NERVE STIMULATION STUDIES

The procedures described in this chapter have their most useful application in those disorders which affect the peripheral nerve, the terminal motor apparatus and its sensory counterpart. Other ENM abnormalities (fibrillations and fasciculations, for example) which play a major role in diagnosis but which are germane to EMG also are found in these diseases. A comprehensive correlation of all ENM studies relative to specific disorders will be found in Chapter 5.

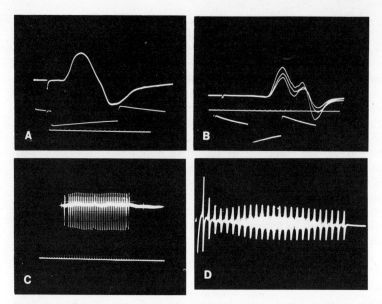

Fig. 2–20. Neuromuscular fatigability recorded during repetitive stimulation. Method I (A and B): Responses to repetitive, supramaximal stimuli delivered at about 3/sec stimulation to median nerve at wrist and recording from thenar muscles. **A.** Normal subject. Upper trace, three superimposed responses; middle trace, calibration, 1 mV; bottom trace, time, 1 msec/division. **B.** Patient with myasthenia gravis. Note progressive decline in amplitude of response with each successive stimulus (upper trace); center trace, 1 msec/division; lower trace, calibration 1 mV. Method II *(C* and *D):* Slow sweep of trace with repetitive supramaximal stimuli at 10–30/sec. Stimulation of right median nerve with recording from thenar muscles. **C.** Normal subject. No decline with repetitive stimuli. **D.** Patient with myasthenia gravis. Note decline in amplitude of compound muscle action potential.

Functional Disorders and Upper Motor Neuron Diseases

In hysteria and malingering, the various parameters are within normal limits. However, the tests which have been described require little or no cooperation on the part of the patient; therefore, the negative result may be quite significant. In patients with upper motor neuron lesions and extrapyramidal disorders, the H reflex is "unmasked" and therefore more easily elicited. Upper motor neuron disorders *per se* show no distinct abnormality of NCV, but the sequellae of paralysis, edema, and vascular changes may produce slight slowing.

Anterior Horn Cell Diseases.

In diseases of the anterior horn cell (motor neuron disease or neuronopathy), conduction velocity usually is within normal limits in the early stages of the disease. However, in advanced stages, when a sufficient number of axons have died, the amplitude of the action potential decreases. Also, as the faster-conducting fibers die, a mild slowing of NCV is not uncommon. On occasion, a mild neuromyal junction defect can be elicited by repetitive stimulation.

Neuropathies

In neuropathies, stimulation studies will be normal until and unless the tested segment has become diseased or affected by remote pathology (i.e., Wallerian degeneration). An example of this is the multiple-root involvement of the Landry–Guillian–Barré syndrome. NSS studies in this disease may be normal if done early in the course of the illness.

The pattern of the neuropathy as detected by NSS assists greatly in differential diagnosis. A distinction between sensory and motor involvement, mono- versus polyneuropathy, and myelin versus axonal involvement (when they can be made) are most helpful clinically.

In those diseases in which myelin primarily is affected, the most striking and characteristic finding is a distinctly slowed NCV. An example is lepromatous neuropathy where the mycobacteria invade the Schwann cell. Further, in this condition, those nerves nearest the skin surface (ulnar and peroneal) are involved earliest and most severely, producing a picture of mononeuritis multiplex. Conditions such as arsenic and uremic poisoning tend to produce lesions of both the axon and the myelin sheath. The pattern here is polyneuropathy, rather than mononeuropathy. In addition to slowing NCV, the amplitude of the compound-muscle-action potential is reduced markedly and its configuration is altered. Perhaps the most common condition in which a striking sensory neuropathy is encountered is diabetes mellitus. The most critical procedure in this case is a sensory conduction study, because involvement of the sensory fibers may precede involvement of the motor fibers by a considerable length of time.

When a peripheral nerve has been severed completely, striking changes are seen. When the lesion is proximal to the stimulation and recording sites, and Wallerian degeneration has not yet occurred, normal or near-normal responses are seen *although function is lost.* There are gradations of slowing as the degeneration progresses. Once Wallerian degeneration has taken place, the fibers are not excitable and no response is seen. When the nerve has been severed completely between the stimulating and recording sites, no response is detected from the outset. As recovery takes place, the nerve becomes excitable *pari passu* with regeneration.

One of the most common conditions in which the latency is prolonged over a specific segment of nerve is the carpal tunnel syndrome. In this condition, the latency obtained by stimulating the median nerve at the wrist and recording from the muscles of the thenar eminence is prolonged. Slowing of the sensory latency of the nerve frequently precedes slowing of the motor latency. Carpal tunnel syndrome occurs as an idiopathic disorder, but also is seen in association with diabetes mellitus, myxedema, rheumatoid arthritis, multiple myeloma, and pregnancy. Other sites of compression of the median nerve have been described which produce specific defects. These include Struthers ligament at the elbow, the anterior interosseous syndrome, and the pronator teres syndrome (35). Entrapment neuropathies of the ulnar, radial, peroneal, and posterior tibial nerves show analogous findings (23).

Neuromyal Junction

The application of conduction studies to disorders of the neuromyal junction has been discussed earlier. A protocol for repetitive stimulation should be tailored to the specific situation.

Myopathies

Nerve stimulation studies usually are within normal limits in the myopathies. The amplitude of the compound-muscle-action potential is diminished if a sufficient number of muscle fibers are nonfunctional; the duration of the action potential may be prolonged and the waveform altered. Abnormalities also may be found with repetitive stimulation studies as described earlier, especially in inflammatory myopathies.

Finally, one must remember that a given disease may affect more than one portion of a peripheral neuromuscular pathway. For example, periarteritis nodosa may affect the peripheral nerve, nerve roots, and muscle in various combinations. In this case, ENM evidence of a neuropathy *and* myopathy will be found. Hypothyroidism is another condition which may produce multiple involvement along the peripheral pathway.

SUMMARY OF STEPS IN PERFORMING NERVE STIMULATION STUDIES.

Step 1. Review all available information regarding the patient, especially the neurologic examination.

Step 2. Introduce yourself to the patient and take him to the room where the test is performed. Perform a neurologic examination, the extent depending upon the clinical situation.

Step 3. Explain the nature of the study to the patient.

Step 4. Turn on all units applicable to the study and see that they are functioning properly.

Step 5. Measure and record the skin temperature over the area to be tested, and cleanse the skin where the electrodes are to be placed with a small amount of alcohol to provide good skin contact.

Step 6. Moisten the recording electrodes with a small amount of electrode paste (jelly) and secure them in position with tape. Insert the electrode wires into the appropriate outlets on the machine, with the active electrode over the belly of the muscle (Fig. 2–2).

Step 7. Place the ground electrode in the appropriate position.

Step 8. Make provision to include the time base and calibration signals in the permanent record for later measurements (Fig. 2–4).

Step 9. Moisten the tips of the stimulating electrode with a small amount of electrode paste. Palpate the nerve at points of intended stimulation. Position the cathode and anode.

Step 10. Start with a small amount of current. Notify the patient when you begin so that he may become accustomed to the sensation. Rapidly reach supramaximal levels and record the trace. Be alert for a myoneural junction defect. If you can see the muscle contract and the patient feels the stimulus, but no trace is seen on the oscilloscope, be certain that the time sweep of the trace is not so fast that the action potential occurs off the screen. This is especially important when the peripheral neuropathy is severe, conduction is markedly slowed, and the response is of low amplitude.

Step 11. Stimulate the nerve at the second point and again record the response to supramaximal stimulation. If measurements are to be made from an auxillary oscilloscope with a persistent image, move the second trace so that the responses are not superimposed (making it difficult to see the shock artifact and onset of response). If repetitive stimulation is to be performed, proceed at this time.

Step 12. Identify the permanent record with the patient's name, the date, the value of the calibration signal, the stimulus duration, and the nerve(s) tested. With a millimeter tape, measure the distance on the skin between the two points of stimulation, cathode-to-cathode, and the distance from the distal point of stimulation to the active electrode. These values should be recorded (Fig. 2–5).

Step 13. From the record, measure the distance from the onset of the first stimulus artifact to the onset of the action potential (initial negative deflection for sensory potentials) (t_1). Calipers may be helpful in making an accurate measurement. Record this interval in msec. Repeat this step for the second point of stimulation (t_2). Subtract t_2 from t_1; the result, t_3, is used to calculate NCV as described earlier:

$$\frac{d}{t_1 - t_2} = \frac{d}{t_3} = \text{m/sec}$$

Measurements of time (msec) are critical and must be made with utmost care because a small error will change the NCV value considerably. When small distances are involved, e.g., across the elbow, the distance measurement also becomes critical. If the preceding value is normal, proceed with further studies as indicated by the nature of the problem. If there is any question as to the result, especially an error in technique, repeat the procedure until you are satisfied that the test is reliable and valid. A comparison with the homologous nerve on the other side is a helpful validation technique.

Step 14. Measure the amplitude of the action potential with calipers from the base line to the highest point of the initial negative (upward) deflection. Using the calipers, compare this height with the calibration signal and convert its value in mV. Measure the duration of the response from the onset of the negative deflection to the end of the response. These values also should be recorded (Fig. 2–5).

Step 15. Upon completion of the study, remove the electrodes carefully; the delicate wires break easily. Cleanse the electrodes and put them in a safe place.

Step 16. After completing the test, it is not wise to go into any detail concerning the findings with the patient. The information is best interpreted to the patient by the clinician in the light of all data available to him, and this should be explained to the patient.

An analogous step-by-step procedure should be followed for sensory conduction studies, H reflex recording, and repetitive stimulation studies.

ARTIFACTS AND SOURCES OF ERROR

Artifacts may be encountered from a variety of sources; some of the more common ones will be discussed. They can be listed as to source and characteristic appearance.

60-Hz Interference

Perhaps the most common artifact and the one which may be most annoying (especially during needle electrode studies described in Ch. 3), is the 60-Hz interference pattern (Fig. 2–21A). It can be recognized by the characteristic highly regular sine-wave trace and by its frequency.

When of low amplitude, it often can be eliminated by use of a suitable filter. When using this filter, one should be aware of the alteration that is made in the time constant and thus in the contour of the traces.

Fig. 2–21.   Artifacts and sources of error. **A.** *1,* 60-cycle interference; *2,* high-frequency feedback; calibration 1 mV, 1 msec/division (lower trace). **B.** Position of recording electrodes reversed; left median nerve stimulated at elbow. *1,* Recording electrode arranged for standard upward negative deflection; *2,* reversal of recording electrodes to the grids. **C.** Large stimulus (shock) artifact; left peroneal nerve stimulated at ankle, recorded from the extensor digitorum brevis; calibration 1 mV. *1,* normal; *2,* large shock artifact produced by poor position of ground electrode. **D.** Polarity of stimulating electrodes reversed; left median nerve stimulated at elbow, recorded from thenar muscle group; calibration 1 mV. Reversal of stimulating cathode and anode (*1,* cathode distal; *2,* cathode proximal) resulted in an additional latency of 0.5 msec. The difference between *1* and *2* represents the time required for the current to traverse the distance between anode and cathode.

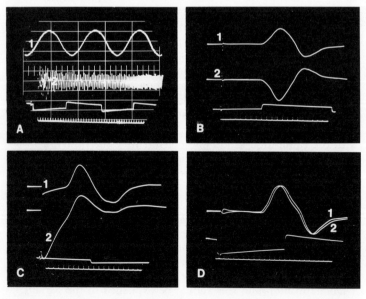

If 60-Hz artifact is present, check the following: 1) equipment ground connections, including equipment–equipment connections; 2) the ground lead on the patient; 3) room lights, especially flourescent, in the immediate vicinity, and outlets to which these lights are connected; 4) equipment used in the immediate vicinity of the room; 5) presence of any broken wires or loose connections, especially those to the patient, and a loose connection to the wall plug; and 6) current leakage. The source of 60-Hz interference often can be identified by test-grounding each item separately.

High-Frequency Feedback

With some equipment, another common but easily correctable artifact results when the audio system volume is excessive. This (signal) produces high-frequency feedback (Fig. 2–21A) which can be eliminated by lowering the volume of the audio system or by housing it in a separate cabinet.

Large Amplitude Stimulus (Shock) Artifact

If the amplitude of the stimulus artifact is unusually large, the ground electrode may be moved to a new position between the stimulating and recording electrodes. By trial and error, the most suitable position for the ground electrode will be found, usually nearer the recording electrode. Sometimes touching the patient with one hand near the recording electrode helps to reduce the amplitude of the shock artifact (Fig. 2–21C). Some machines contain a circuit to reduce the size of the shock artifact (1).

No Recordable Action Potential

If the muscle can be seen to contract but no action potential registers on the screen, one or more of the following may be the cause:

1. The recording electrodes are not plugged into the machine.
2. The electrodes, especially the one over the muscle, have not been secured properly or have loosened and/or fallen off entirely.
3. The recording electrode wires are broken.
4. The sensitivity setting is insufficient to detect the action potential (See Step 10, this chapter).
5. Subcutaneous edema is present. Subcutaneous edema may increase the resistance between muscle and recording electrode to the point where, despite muscular contraction, no action potential is recorded. Under such circumstances, needle electrodes should be used for recording and, if necessary, for stimulation. With the latter, the stimulus intensity can be reduced. These electrodes can be inserted in proximity to the nerve and muscle, respectively.
6. The time base selected does not match the latency of response. When the latter is prolonged, the action potential is "off the screen." A longer time base should be employed.

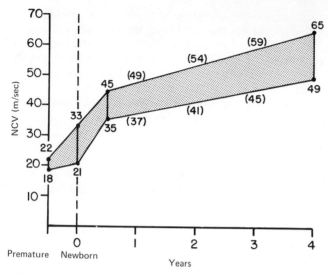

Fig. 2–22.   Relationship between age and NCV (ulnar nerve). Illustration of the relationship between chronological age and NCV (in m/sec.). The data are extrapolated from Thomas and Lambert, 1960. The rate of increase is 2–3 m/sec every 6 months over the range of 6 months to 4 years, at which time adult range is achieved.

Reversal of Polarity

If the polarity of the action potential is reversed from that usually observed, the recording electrodes may not be plugged into the machine properly. The contour and amplitude of the action potential may vary with the position and size of the recording electrodes. Maximum amplitude and initial negative deflection are produced when the active electrode is directly over the end-plate region. When the response to stimulation of a nerve does not appear with an initial negative deflection, the position and polarity of the electrodes should be reversed.

Reversing the stimulating anode and cathode will cause an error in the measured time value; the cathode always should be in apposition to the recording electrode (Fig. 2–21B). In dealing with infants and small children, take great care to place the electrodes before proceeding with stimulation because only a few stimuli can be delivered before the patient may cease to cooperate.

Crossover Phenomenon (Martin–Gruber Anastomosis)

A variation which may be encountered on stimulation of the median and ulnar nerves is called "the crossover phenomenon." In some normal individuals, nerve fibers to the muscles of the thenar eminence that lie in the median nerve at the elbow travel in the ulnar nerve at this level. Distal to this point in the forearm, the fibers cross over to the median nerve. When this situation is present, supramaximal stimulation of the median nerve at the elbow elicits an action potential of small amplitude compared with that obtained when the nerve is stimulated at the wrist.

Table 2-1. NORMAL VALUES FOR NERVE STIMULATION STUDIES

Motor Nerve Conduction Velocity		
Nerve	Normal Range (msec)	Reference
Ulnal		
elbow–wrist	49.0–65.6	Thomas et al, 1959 (40)
axilla–elbow	50.0–73.9	Gilliatt and Thomas, 1960 (17)
Median		
elbow–wrist	48.3–67.9	Thomas, 1960 (39)
axilla–elbow	47.8–69.6	Thomas, 1960 (39)
Peroneal	43.3–57.8	Carpendale, 1956 (5)
Posterior tibial	41.9–55.3	Mavor and Atcheson, 1966 (28)
Sciatic (to medial head of gastrocnemius)	45.0–60.0	Yap and Hirota, 1967 (44)
Radial (to brachioradialis)	72.4–75.6	Gassel and Diamantopoulos, 1964 (15)

Nerve Conduction Times			
SENSORY			
Nerve	Distance (cm)	Normal Range (msec)	Reference
Ulnar	10–13	2.1–3.0	
Medial	10–13	2.3–3.2	
Peroneal		4.7–7.1	Mawdsley and Mayer, 1965 (30)
Posterior tibial		6.1–8.1	Mawdsley and Mayer, 1965 (30)
MOTOR			
Ulnar	10–13	2.3–3.4	Mavor and Libman, 1962 (29)
Median	10–13	2.7–4.2	Mavor and Libman, 1962 (29)
Peroneal		3.7–6.1	Carpendale, 1956 (5)
Posterior tibial		4.2–6.7	Mavor and Atcheson, 1966 (28)
Radial	18	4.2–7.1	Downie and Scott, 1964 (9)
Brachial plexus to			
Deltoid	15–19	4.2–4.5	Gassel, 1965 (15)
Biceps brachii	19–29	4.5–5.1	
Tripceps brachii	20–30	4.4–4.6	
Supraspinatus	8–11	2.5–2.8	
Infraspinatus	13–18	3.3–3.5	
Facial	10–11	2.7–4.0	Langworth and Taverner, 1963 (25)
Femoral	14–16	3.9–5.0	Gassel, 1964 (15)

That this is due to crossover may be verified by stimulating the ulnar nerve at the elbow and recording a compound-muscle-action potential from the thenar eminence. The sum of the amplitudes of the two responses (obtained by stimulating the median and ulnar nerves at the elbow) is approximately equal to the response obtained when only the median nerve is stimulated at the wrist.

"N" Potential

A potential which sometimes is detected and has been confused with a compound-muscle-action potential has been described under various names, the "n" potential, the nerve action potential, or the intramuscular nerve action potential (33). It is seen most frequently when motor nerves are stimulated at the wrist (Fig. 2–16C). Its amplitude is an extremely small 5–20 μV compared with the compound-muscle-action potential of about 1–5 mV. It is detected only with high-sensitivity-gain settings when an active needle electrode is in the end-plate zone or an active surface electrode is over it. It has an initial negative deflection and a latency of 1–2 msec when the distance is 6–9 cm. This potential appears to originate from intramuscular motor nerve fibers in the end-plate zone (3). Failure to recognize the "n" potential produces erroneous latency and conduction velocity measurements of the motor nerve.

Temperature of the Extremity and Age of the Patient

Conduction velocity will vary with neuromuscular temperature; the variation is especially significant in the more superficial nerves. The relationship of conduction to temperature is direct, about a 2.5 m/sec decrease for every degree centigrade over a limited range (29–38°C) (8). This factor should be borne in mind, especially when a slightly slow NCV is found. Conduction velocity also varies with age (Fig. 2–22). It is much slower in infants than in adults. Adult values are usually attained by 3–5 years (38, 43).

Miscellaneous

Other sources of error in nerve conduction studies have been described (14, 33). These include 1) anomalous innervation of the muscles, 2) potentials detected from muscles which are at a distance from the recording electrodes, and 3) spread of the stimulus to a nerve other than that to which the stimulus is delivered ("crosstalk").

NORMAL VALUES

Table 2–1 lists normal values of various parameters for different nerves. Each diagnostic center should establish its own values by adequate study of normal subjects. A number of such values has been published (37) but they vary somewhat from laboratory to laboratory. Among the reasons for this variation are lack of control of extremity temperature (probably the most significant variable), the general health of the control subjects (prediabetics, unsuspected systemic disorders, and debilitating diseases), and the ages of the control subjects. Some laboratories separate normal values into age groups, even within the adult range. This is important in dealing with older populations where there normally is some slowing of NCV. Finally, there are technical factors: accuracy and design of equipment used, and the care taken with measurements and placement of electrodes.

The extremes of the normal range are uncertain, especially at the lower end of the scale. When there is some question as to the response of a particular nerve, a control study of the homologous nerve on the opposite side of the body should be performed.

REFERENCES

1. Andersen VO, Buchtal F: Low noise a.c. amplifier and compensator to reduce stimulus artifact. Med Biol Eng 8: 501–508, 1970
2. Blom S, Finnstrom O: Motor conduction velocities in newborn infants of various gestational ages. Acta Paediatr Scand 57: 377–384, 1968
2a. Brandstater ME, Dinsdale SM: Electrophysiological Studies in the Assessment of Spinal Cord Lesions. Arch Phys Med Rehabil 57: 70–74, 1976
3. Buchtal F, Rosenfalck P: Evoked action potentials and conduction velocity in human sensory nerves. Brain Res 3 (1): 122, 1966 (Special Issue)
4. Buchtal F, Rosenfalck P: Sensory potentials in polyneuropathy. Brain 94: 241–262, 1971
5. Carpendale MIF: Conduction time in the terminal portion of the motor fibers of ulnar, median and peroneal nerves in healthy subjects and in patients with neuropathy. University of Minnesota, Unpublished Master's Thesis, 1956
6. Casey EB, LeQuesne PM: Digital nerve action potentials in healthy subjects and in carpal tunnel and diabetic patients. J Neurol Neurosurg Psychiatry 35: 612–623, 1972
7. Dawson GD, Merton PA: Recurrent discharges from motorneurons (abstr). Bruxelles, 2nd Int Congr Physiol Sci, 1956, pp 221–222
8. DeJesus PV, Hausmanowa–Petrusewicz I, Banchi RL: The effect of cold on nerve conduction of human's slow and fast nerve fibers. Neurology (Minneap) 23: 1182–1189, 1973
9. Downie AW, Scott TR: Radial nerve conduction studies. Neurology (Minneap) 14: 839, 1964
9a. Dyck PJ, Lais AC, Ohta M, Bastion JA, Okazaki H, Groover RV: Chronic Inflammatory Polyradiculoneuropathy. Mayo Clin Proc 50: 621–637, 1975
10. Ekstedt J: Human single muscle fibre action potentials. Acta Physiol Scand 61 [Suppl 226]: 1–91, 1964
11. Ekstedt J, Stalberg E: Single fiber electromyography for the study of the microphysiology of the human muscle. In Desmedt JE (ed): New Developments in Electromyography and Clinical Neurophysiology, Vol I. Basel, Karger, 1973, pp 89–112
12. Erlanger J, Gasser H: Electrical signs of nervous activity. Philadelphia, University of Pennsylvania Press, 1937, p 221
13. Fullerton PM: The effect of ischemia on nerve conduction in the carpal tunnel syndrome. J Neurol Neurosurg Psychiatry 26: 385–397, 1963
14. Gassel MM: Sources of error in motor nerve conduction studies. Neurology (Minneap) 14: 825, 1964
15. Gassel MM, Diamantopoulos E: Pattern of conduction times in the distribution of the radial nerve. Neurology (Minneap) 14: 222, 1964
16. Gassel MM, Trojaborg WJ: Clinical and electrophysiological study of the pattern of conduction times in the distribution of the sciatic nerve. J Neurol Neurosurg Psychiatry 27: 351, 1964
17. Gilliatt RW, Thomas PK: Changes in nerve conduction with ulnar lesions at the elbow. J Neurol Neurosurg Psychiatry 23: 312, 1960
18. Hodes R, Larabee MG, German W: The human electromyogram in response to nerve stimulation and the conduction velocity of motor axons: studies on normal and on injured peripheral nerves. Arch Neurol Psychiat (Chicago) 60: 340–365, 1948
19. Hoffmann PP: Versuche uber Bahnung und Hemmurng im menschlichen Ruckenmark. Med Klin 16: 673, 1920
20. Hoffmann P: Untersuchung uber die Eigenreflexe (Schneureflexe) menschlichen Muskeln. Berlin, Springer, 1922, p 106

21. Johns RJ, Grob D, Harvey AM: Studies in neuromuscular function II. Effects of nerve stimulation in normal subjects and in patients with myasthenia gravis. Johns Hopkins Med J 99: 125, 1956

22. Kimura J: F-wave velocity in the central segment of the median and ulnar nerve. Neurology (Minneap) 24: 539–546, 1974

22a. Kimura J, Bosch P, Lindsay GM: F-Wave Conduction Velocity in the Central Segment of the Peroneal and Tibial Nerves. Arch Phys Med Rehabil 56: 492–497, 1975

23. Koppell HP, Thompson WAL: Peripheral Entrapment Neuropathies. Baltimore, William & Wilkins, 1963, p 171

24. Lambert EH, Rooke EB, Eaton LM, Hodgson CH: Myasthenic syndrome occasionally associated with bronchial neoplasm: neurophysiological studies in myasthenia gravis. In Viets H (ed): Springfield, Ill, CC Thomas, 1961, pp 362–410

25. Langworth EP, Taverner D: The prognosis in facial palsy. Brain 86: 465, 1963

25a. London GW: Normal ulnar nerve conduction velocity across the thoracic outlet: comparison of two measuring techniques. J Neurol Neurosurg Psychiatry 38: 756–760, 1975

26. Lovelace RE, Myers SJ, Zablow L: Sensory conduction in peroneal and posterior tibial nerves using averaging techniques. J Neurol Neurosurg Psychiatry 36: 942–950, 1973

27. Magladery JW, McDougall DB: Electrophysiological studies of nerve and reflex activity in normal man. Johns Hopkins Med J 86: 265, 1950

28. Mavor H, Atcheson JB: Posterior tibial nerve conduction: velocity of sensory and motor fibers. Arch Neurol 14: 661, 1966

29. Mavor H, Libman I: Motor nerve conduction velocity measurement as a diagnostic tool. Neurology (Minneap) 12: 733, 1962

30. Mawdsley C, Mayer RF: Nerve conduction in alcoholic polyneuropathy. Brain 88: 335, 1965

31. Ozdemic C, Young RR: Electrical testing in myasthenia gravis. Ann NY Acad Sci 181: 287–302, 1971

32. Ruskin P, Rogoff JB: Simultaneous sensory and motor nerve conduction latency noting effect of topical anesthesia. Arch Phys Med Rehabil 45: 597, 1964

33. Simpson JA: Fact and fallacy in measurement of conduction velocity in motor nerves. J Neurol Neurosurg Psychiatry 27: 381, 1964

34. Simpson JA: Disorders of neuromuscular transmission. Proc R Soc Med 59: 993–998, 1966

35. Smith RV, Fisher RG: Struthers ligament: a source of median nerve compression above the elbow. J Neurosurg 38: 778–779, 1973

35a. Stalberg E: Single Fiber Electromyography. Herlev, Denmark, Disa Information Department, Disa Electonics, 1974, p 20

36. Stalberg E, Ekstedt J: Single fibre EMG and microphysiology of the motor unit in normal and diseased human muscle. In Desmedt JE (ed): New Developments in Electromyography and Clinical Neurophysiology, Vol I. Basel, Karger, 1973, pp 113–129

37. Sunderland S: Nerves and Nerve Injuries. London, E & S Livingstone, 1968, pp 277–280; 386–388

37a. Thiele B, Stalberg E: Single fibre EMG findings in polyneuropathies of different aetiology. J Neurol Neurosurg Psychiatry 38: 881–887, 1975

38. Thomas PK: Motor nerve conduction in the carpal tunnel syndrome. Neurology (Minneap) 10: 1045, 1960

39. Thomas JE, Lambert EH: Ulnar nerve conduction velocity and H-reflex in infants and children. J Appl Physiol 15: 1, 1960

40. Thomas PK, Sears TA, Gilliatt RW: The range of conduction velocity in normal motor nerve fibers to the small muscles of the hand and foot. J Neurol Neurosurg Psychiatry 22: 175, 1959

41. Thorne J: Central responses to electrical activation of the peripheral nerves supplying the intrinsic hand muscles. J Neurol Neurosurg Psychiatry 28: 482–495, 1965

42. Wager EW Jr, Buerger AA: A linear relationship between H-reflex latency and sensory conduction velocity in diabetic neuropathy. Neurology (Minneap) 24: 711–714, 1974

43. Wagner AL, Buchtal F: Motor and sensory conduction in infancy and childhood. Dev Med Child Neurol 14: 189–216, 1972

44. Yap CB, Hirota T: Sciatic nerve motor conduction velocity study. J Neurol Neurosurg Psychiatry 30: 233, 1967

three

NEEDLE ELECTRODE STUDIES: ELECTROMYOGRAPHY

INTRODUCTION

The technique of EMG is used to study the electrical activity within a muscle. This is accomplished by inserting a needle electrode into it. The electrical activity detected at the needle is circuited to an amplifier and displayed on an oscilloscope and over a loudspeaker. The characteristics of the discharges are analyzed from these modalities (as well as by more sophisticated techniques described later).

In 1929, Adrian and Bronk (1) first demonstrated the value of this method. The comprehensive study of Weddel, Feinstein, and Pattle (21) indicated the significance of this technique in normal and pathologic states. Numerous studies have followed, defining the abnormalities in systemic disorders, motor neuron disease, pathologic states of the peripheral nerve, myoneural junction disorders, and myopathies.

The following discussion includes a description of EMG techniques, and the parameters of the various types of normal and abnormal electrical activity.

TECHNIQUE

The necessary equipment is described in Chapter 1. Several varieties of needle electrodes are available. Their capabilities differ with their electrical characteristics. Most electroneuromyographers employ one or two types of needles and are familiar with their limitations. *Monopolar* needles may be used for all varieties of muscle exploration and are especially useful in examining small muscles (extraocular, facial, and small muscles of the hand). One of the *bipolar* types, concentric or coaxial (bifilar), is practical for general use and obviates the need for a second grid in the form of another needle or a surface metal plate electrode (Fig. 3–5). If, during the test, the needle touches the table or some contaminated area, another sterile

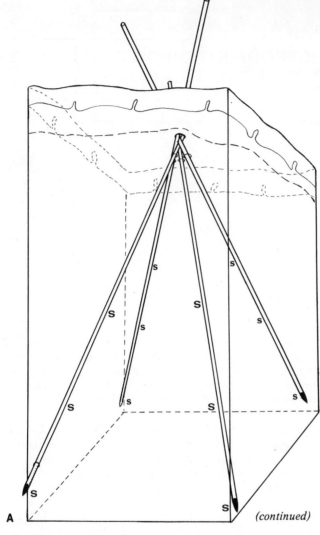

A   *(continued)*

Fig. 3–1. "Quadrant" technique for needle electrode studies. **A.** Diagram showing a needle electrode inserted four times (represented by four needles), once in each quadrant, sampling three successive depths at each site. **B.** Photomicrograph of muscle biopsy with coaxial needle electrode placed on slide in apposition to muscle showing relative sizes of electrode and muscle fibers as well as area subtended by needle tip.

needle must be used. The needle should not be placed on a table or in some location where it may be dulled or bent.

During the procedure, a ground electrode is placed on the patient's body and secured with a rubber strap or tape. Generally, the ground electrode may be left

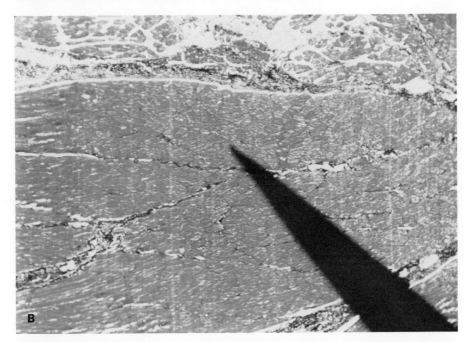

Fig. 3–1 B.

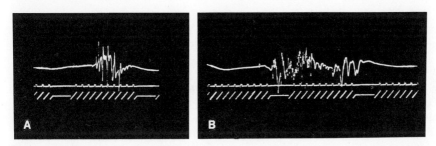

Fig. 3–2.   Insertion activity recorded with a monopolar needle electrode. **A.** Burst from normal muscle. **B.** A prolonged burst from a partially denervated muscle. Calibration, 100 μV. Time, 10 msec/staircase.

in place while the needle electrode is moved from muscle to muscle (if the ground and needle electrodes are on opposite sides of the body, electrocardiac (ECG) artifact may contaminate the recording).

The simplest method to *display* EMG potentials, and the one most commonly employed, is the "watch-listen" technique. Although unsophisticated, this method has the advantage of immediate evaluation of a large number of potentials because of its simplicity. It is excellent for scanning relatively large areas of tissue. For more detailed quantitative analysis, especially of abnormal potentials, other forms of more permanent display are used: 1) persistent fluorescent cathode; 2) still photographs; 3) motion pictures; 4) ultraviolet or metallic paper

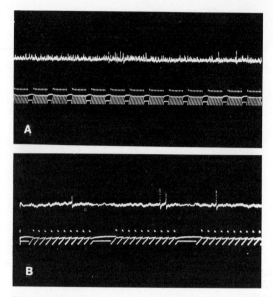

Fig. 3–3. End-plate noise and miniature end-plate potentials. **A.** End-plate noise recorded from the left gastrocnemius muscle at rest. Note the numerous small discharges (MEPPs?). These disappear when the needle is moved a short distance. **B.** Small action potentials recorded from paraspinal muscles at rest. These are either miniature end-plate potentials or small intramuscular nerve-fiber-action potentials. Calibration, 10 μV. Time, 10 msec/staircase. Monopolar needle electrode.

recording systems; and 5) magnetic tape recording. The use of signal delay has the advantage of on-line viewing of individual potentials, single fiber potentials, and for jitter studies (9). Each method can be used individually or in combination; they permit storage of information for analysis at the examiner's discretion, and documentation as part of a permanent record. Still more elaborate methods involve analysis by computer techniques, either on-line or by replay from magnetic tape. Computer methods are not yet in routine use. Their clinical application for various disorders is being assessed. Improved techniques well may alter the current status.

SITES FOR TESTING

There is no simple routine, no single blueprint indicating which muscles to test. As with other ENM studies, knowledge of the patient's history and physical findings is a prerequisite for EMG. This will determine a most important decision of the EMG examination: which muscle or muscles to test.

For example, in a patient suspected of having amyotrophic lateral sclerosis, several muscles in each extremity should be studied. At times, a lesion of the brachial plexus can be differentiated from a multiple root lesion even though a similar pattern of denervation may be seen in the muscles of the affected limb in both. The root lesion may involve the paraspinal muscles supplied by the posterior primary rami, whereas the plexus lesion will not.

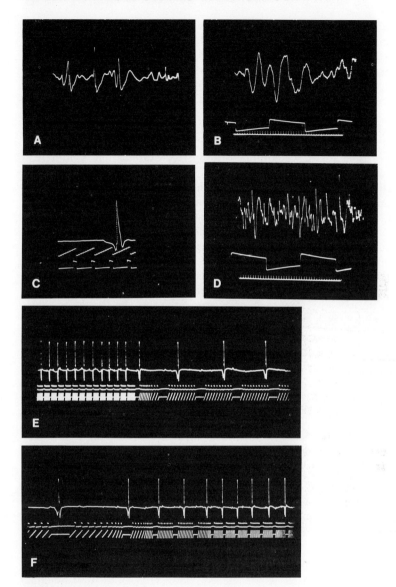

Fig. 3–4. Normal motor unit potentials (MUPs). **A.** Individual MUPs in close proximity to needle tip (rounded potentials are distant); monopolar needle recording from left first dorsal interosseus muscle, normal subject; calibration (B) 1 mV, 1 msec/per division. **B.** Individual, distant MUP; recording identical with *A* and taken immediately thereafter by moving needle tip; calibration 200 μV, 1 msec/division. **C.** Normal MUP recorded from the right biceps muscle, coaxial needle electrode; minimum voluntary contraction; calibration, 500 μV. **D.** Ocular muscle MUP; monopolar recording from left lateral rectus, normal subject; calibration, 200 μV, 1 msec/division. **E. F.** Repetitively firing, single, normal MUP from the right internal hamstring muscle, shown at several sweep speeds; calibration, 100 μV; time 10 msec/staircase; monopolar needle electrode.

If a lumbar disc is thought to be the causative lesion, the presence of single- or multiple-root involvement must be determined. In myasthenia gravis, more information is gained from examining the clinically affected muscles. In the instance of a myopathy, examination of proximal and distal muscles will help establish the pattern of disease and its degree. Much of the value of EMG is lost and the patient unnecessarily exhausted (or put to stress) when only inappropriate muscles are examined.

The nature of the study should be briefly explained to the patient so that he will know what to expect. Greater cooperation is required from the patient for needle electrode studies than for nerve stimulation or EDX examination. Children in particular can be difficult to study.

When a particular muscle is tested, the needle should be moved so that different areas within one muscle are sampled. The habit of sampling in several directions and depths must be developed. An adequate sampling can be made using the "four-quadrant" technique (Fig. 3–1). The needle should be inserted into the belly of the muscle perpendicular to the skin with a swift, smooth motion. The electrical activity of the muscle is studied under several conditions: 1) on insertion or movement of the needle; 2) with the muscle relaxed; and 3) with varying degrees of voluntary contraction. In some cases, it is well to record the discharges as they occur and review them at leisure. Each test site should be examined carefully under each condition: rest, voluntary contraction, and needle movement.

NORMAL POTENTIALS

Activity on Insertion and Needle Movement

On insertion or movement of the needle, a brief burst of electrical activity occurs (Fig. 3–2). It lasts less than one sec and generally is 50–250 μV in amplitude. These insertion potentials produce a characteristic "burrrrr" sound, like a brief scratch of a needle on a phonograph record. This activity, recurring each time the needle is moved, probably is produced by direct irritation of the muscle fibers.

Activity at Rest

Under normal circumstances, with the needle at rest and the muscle relaxed, no electrical activity is discernable; only the background noise of the equipment can be heard and seen. If the muscle is not relaxed completely, motor unit potential activity will be present. This is especially common in muscles that have a high degree of "tonicity," e.g., the external anal sphincter and the paraspinal muscles (6). If relaxation is incomplete, the patient should be instructed to relax the muscle ("let the extremity go limp") or the examiner may have to reposition the patient and/or the extremity. Under two circumstances, however, potentials can be detected with the muscle truly at rest and may be confused with abnormal potentials.

Occasionally the tip of the needle may touch a nerve twig, and electrical activity from it will be detected. These potentials are of low amplitude, usually less than 150–200 μV, and of short duration, less than 3 msec. They fire repetitively, 10–20/second. They disappear promptly when the needle is moved a short distance.

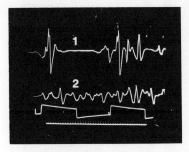

Fig. 3–5. Monopolar *(1)* and coaxial *(2)* needle recordings of MUP from right tibialis anterior with both needles in close proximity at the same site; recorded simultaneously on two channels during minimal voluntary contraction; calibration, 1 mV, 1 msec/division.

Abnormal spontaneous activity, positive waves, and especially fibrillations, must be distinguished from nerve action potentials.

The needle tip also may encounter the motor end-plate region and detect *"end-plate noise"* (Fig. 3–3).

On the oscilloscope screen, the amplitude of the baseline increases persistently and a soft blowing noise is heard over the speaker. Individual potentials with the characteristics of *miniature end-plate potentials* sometimes are encountered. These show an initial negative deflection, are 0.5–2 msec in duration and 20–100 μV in amplitude. They are superimposed on the enlarged baseline ("blowing noise"). These also resemble the action potentials of intramuscular nerve fibers. This activity is lost easily with slight movement of the needle. Both nerve action potentials and end-plate noise may be confused with abnormal potentials at rest.

Activity on Muscle Contraction

On voluntary contraction, motor unit potentials (MUPs) appear (Fig. 3–4, 3–5). The term *motor unit* refers to the anatomic composite of anterior horn cell body and its appendages, the axon, the neuromyal junction, and the muscle fibers (cells) innervated by the axon twigs of that neuron. The innervation ratio (number of muscle cells supplied by one neuron via its axon) and fiber type vary with each muscle. The innervation ratio, the size of the muscle fibers, and their territory account for variation in amplitude, duration, and waveform of MUPs. *Motor unit potentials,* then, are the electrical discharges produced by voluntary contraction of the muscle. They represent the changes in the electrical field over the surface of the muscle cell.

A MUP is the prelude to the mechanical contraction process which occurs about 0.5 msec later. The parameters of the MUP—size (amplitude), duration, shape (mono-, di-, tri-, polyphasic), and frequency of firing—vary with a number of factors, some of which are unknown.

The size of the individual muscle fibers within a motor unit is a major factor determining the amplitude and duration of the MUP. For example, the MUPs of the extrinsic eye muscles are extremely small and easily can be mistaken for fibrillation potentials; those of the triceps muscle are among the largest MUPs which occur under normal circumstances.

However, the size of the muscle fibers is not the only determinant of amplitude and duration. The MUPs of the first dorsal interosseous muscle, for example, are far from small and not commensurate with the size of the muscle fibers in that

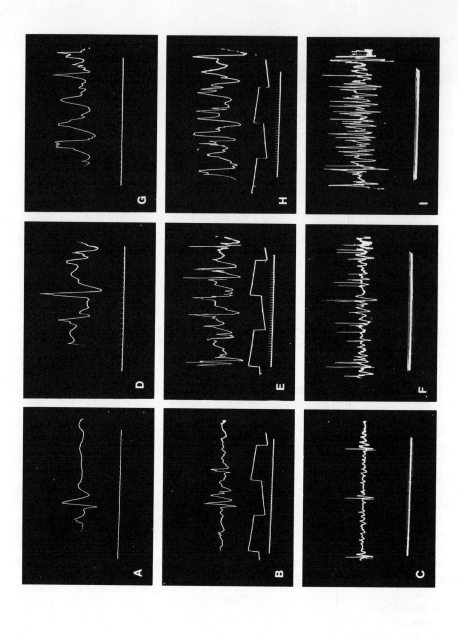

◀ **Fig. 3–6.** Interference patterns produced by increasing strength of muscle contraction and displayed at varying sweep speeds. All recordings were taken from left first dorsal interosseus muscle of the same patient at one sitting; calibration, 1 mV, 1 msec/division. **A. B. C.** No interference (discrete MUP), minimum recruitment. **D. E. F.** Mixed interference pattern, partial recruitment. **G. H. I.** Full interference pattern, maximum recruitment.

Sweep speed (msec/cm)	Interference pattern		
	None	Mixed	Full
5	A	D	G
10	B	E	H
30	C	F	I

muscle. These parameters as well as shape (waveform) may be related to another variable, namely the distribution of the muscle fibers of one motor unit within the muscle. Brandstater and Lambert (2) have described a random distribution of the fibers of a motor unit. They may be dispersed over as much as 12% of the muscle diameter; furthermore, not all the fibers in a single motor unit lie within one fascicle. The frequency of firing of MUPs has been studied extensively and may be related to a number of factors (15)—fiber type, impulse rate, and physiologic state of the muscle fiber.

Some electrical characteristics of individual fiber types may be distinguished in normal cooperative patients and in certain disease states (11).

With the needle electrode in the muscle and on voluntary contraction, the clarity with which the MUPs are heard and seen varies with the proximity of the tip of the needle to the motor end-plate. If the MUPs sound distant or muffled and have a rounded contour, the needle tip is not close enough to those units. Careful movement of the needle will bring the tip closer to the "generator site," as evidenced by larger and more distinct MUPs that also sound "sharper and clearer." Measurement of amplitude and duration never should be made if the MUPs are dull and muted with a rounded contour. The needle should be moved until the MUPs no longer are "distant," but clear both visually and audibly.

The strength of contraction determines the number of motor units and, therefore, the number of MUPs brought into play (*recruitment* of MUP) (Fig. 3–6). With a sustained but *minimal contraction,* one or more MUPs will be seen to fire repetitively. When two or three units are firing, they may be distinguished one from the other by their parameters: amplitude, duration, shape, and firing rate.

During minimal contraction, the following parameters of the MUPs should be observed: 1) amplitude of each MUP (mV or μV); 2) duration (msec); 3) waveform or shape (mono-, di-, tri-, or polyphasic); 4) rate of firing; 5) alteration of firing rate with slight increase in strength of contraction; 6) the introduction of additional units into the firing pattern with increasing strength of contraction; 7) the number of MUP units relative to the strength of contraction; and 8) the pattern of activity on cessation of contraction.

Maximal contraction produces a distinct pattern with a typical sound. It has been referred to as a *mixed* or *interference pattern,* to describe the overlap as each of a number of units fires at its own frequency. Individual adjacent MUPs fuse and cannot be identified during this phase of testing. The exact appearance of this

Table 3-1. CHARACTERISTICS OF EMG POTENTIALS

Potential	Amplitude (μv)	Duration (msec)	Wave form (-phasic)
A. Normal			
1. MUP	500–3000	2–10	Di or tri
2. Polyphasic	50–3000	2–25	Poly (5–25)
3. Nerve	20–240	1–4	Di
B. Abnormal			
1. MUP			
(a) "Giant"	3000–10,000	5–30	Di or tri
(b) "Myopathic"	50–500	1–6	Di or tri
(c)Doublets–triplets	500–3000	2–10	Di or tri
2. Resting			
(a) Fibrillation	10–100	1–2	Mono or di
(b) Fasciculation	50–500	2–10	Di, tri or poly
(c) Positive sharp waves	Variable	Up to 100	Di

pattern on the oscilloscope screen is a function of the sweep speed (Fig. 3–6).

The number of MUPs produced by *maximal contraction* can be reported by using a simple scale of $0-3+$: 0 corresponds to "no potentials noted", $1+$ indicates that only single, isolated MUPs are produced; $2+$ indicates that more than single MUPs are produced, but the oscilloscope screen is not "full"; and $3+$ implies a full interference pattern so that potentials overlap each other continuously.

PARAMETERS OF NORMAL MOTOR UNIT POTENTIALS   Together with other measurements, Table 3–1 lists the parameters of MUPs. These potentials produced by voluntary contraction should not be confused with the compound-muscle-action potentials elicited during nerve stimulation studies, which are evoked responses. In the muscles of the extremities, MUP generally are 5–10 msec in duration, 0.5–2 mV in amplitude, and are bi- or triphasic. The firing frequency is 5–20/sec. With the needle stationary and with a weak sustained contraction, the parameters remain constant for that MUP; i.e., there is no appreciable variation in amplitude, duration, and waveform.

Motor unit potentials of certain muscles have unique characteristics which differ widely from others, and the electroneuromyographer must become familiar with them. The small MUPs of facial muscles would be considered abnormal if recorded in the triceps muscle. Normally, less than 5–8% of the MUP sampled in a muscle are *polyphasic* (Fig. 3–7). When the examiner has the impression that the percentage of polyphasic MUPs is increased, a permanent record should be made for a quantitative assessment.

The parameters of a polyphasic potential can be quite variable. One unique type of polyphasic potential consists of a burst followed by a brief silent period and then a small bi- or triphasic potential. This small MUP following the large burst has been referred to as "parasite" (7), "pony potential," or "coupled discharge" (Fig. 3–9D). These potentials may be related to slowly conducting nerve sprouts (16).

Frequency (no./sec.	Sound	Remarks
Up to 500	Low-pitched machine gun	
2–30	Rough, rasping, rattling	Under 5% of voluntary potentials
3–150	High-pitched machine gun	
Few	Loud machine gun	Few potentials relative to strength of contraction
Many	High-pitched rapid firing	Many potentials relative to strength of contraction
2–30	Wrinkling cellophane (high-pitched click)	
2–20	Typing on cardboard (dull thud)	
2–100	High-pitched crackling	

While a slight variation in the number of polyphasic MUPs is in itself of no great clinical significance, a definite increase coupled with the presence of other abnormalities is of great importance.

ABNORMAL POTENTIALS

In this section, two varieties of abnormalities will be discussed: 1) abnormal variations of normally encountered potentials; and 2) potentials not encountered in *most* normal states. This latter qualification is necessary because some of the potentials to be described may be present at times without clear clinical significance. One should be certain before labelling a potential as abnormal, assess its parameters carefully, and be sure that it occurs more than just once or twice in the course of testing. Is it an artifact? Is it related to a state of incomplete relaxation?

Abnormal Variations of Normal Potentials

INSERTION POTENTIALS   When there is significant muscle atrophy, and the number of electrically excitable muscle fibers *diminishes,* the duration of *normal* insertion activity declines proportionately. This is also the case in the initial period following nerve transection. With complete atrophy, such insertion activity is *absent.* This is also the case in the acute phase of familial periodic paralysis.

Insertion of the needle can evoke a number of *abnormal* potentials: fibrillation, positive waves, myotonic discharges, etc. We refer to this phenomenon as *"increased" insertion* activity (called "increased irritability" by some authors).

END-PLATE NOISE   No distinct abnormality of this phenomenon has been correlated with a clinical syndrome, even though the motor end-plate has been described as enlarged in some diseases.

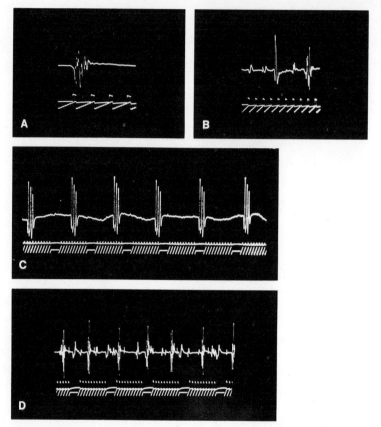

Fig. 3–7. Polyphasic MUP. **A.** Polyphasic MUP recorded from the tibialis anterior, minimum voluntary contraction, coaxial needle electrode; calibration, 1 mV, 10 msec/"staircase" in all figures. **B.** Triphasic followed by polyphasic MUP recorded from the same muscle. Note distant MUP. Recording condition as in *A.* **C.** Repetitively firing polyphasic MUP from same muscle with weak contraction; calibration, 100 μV. **D.** Overlapping of poly- and triphasic MUP firing repetitively; calibration, 100 μV.

MOTOR UNIT POTENTIALS   MUP abnormalities consist of alterations of amplitude, duration, frequency, waveform, number, and grouping. The mechanism of some of the abnormal parameters of MUPs is shown in Fig. 3–8.

In diseases of the anterior horn cell, the amplitude and duration of the MUPs increase. These alterations are ascertained from the oscilloscope screen and by means of permanent recording for accurate measurements. These large, so-called "giant" action potentials exceed 5 mV in amplitude (Fig. 3–9A). As the motor neuron disease progresses, the number of remaining motor units decreases and there is a consequent decrease in the number of MUPs. The interference pattern eventually shows single, isolated motor units with a loss of overlap of MUPs, i.e., the interference pattern is reduced; the rate of firing is decreased. MUP territory studies indicate an increase in the area of each active unit. There is also an increase in the duration of each MUP, with some increase in polyphasic potentials.

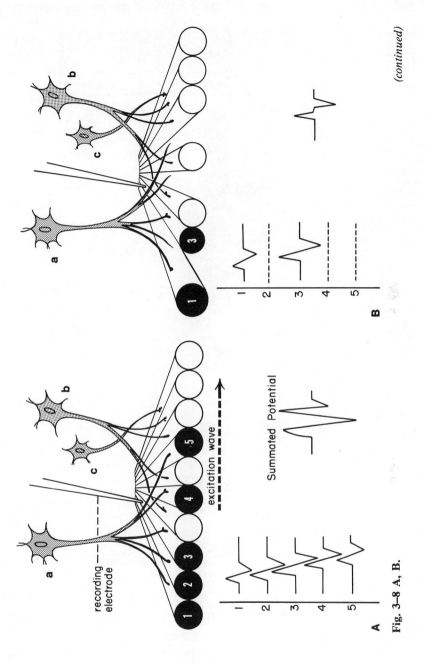

Fig. 3–8 A, B.

(continued)

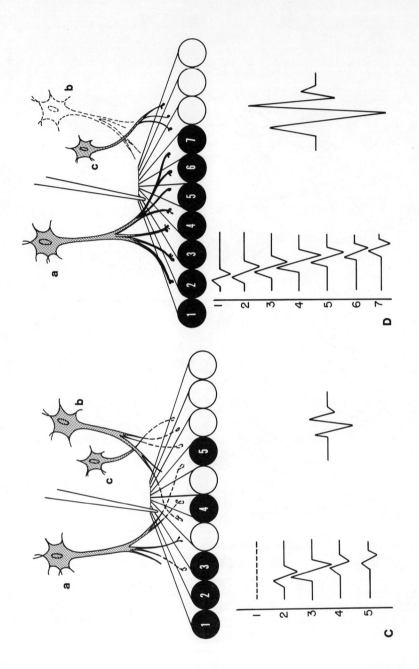

◄ **Fig. 3–8.** MUP—the mechanism of normal and abnormal EMG waveform production. For each condition (*A.* Normal. *B.* Myopathy. *C.* Neuropathy. *D.* Neuronopathy), three motor units are depicted diagrammatically. Anterior horn cells *a, b,* and *c* send axons peripherally to innervate a group of muscle fibers depicted as cylinders. Of the 10 muscle fibers shown, only those subserved by motorneuron *A* have been numbered *(1* through *5).* **A.** When Cell a fires, the excitation wave sweeps from left to right, causing fibers *1* through *5* to fire in sequence. The action potentials of the individual muscle fibers are shown in vertical projection at the lower left corner of each diagram. The potential of each fiber begins slightly later than the preceding one because of the spatial dispersion of the motor unit in reference to the wave of excitation. Because recording EMG needle electrode is over fiber *3,* the amplitude of this fiber's action potential will be the largest of the series; that of fibers *2* and *4* will be less; and fibers *1* and *5* will have the smallest amplitude of all. The EMG recording needle will register a summated potential which is made up of the individual muscle fiber potentials as they are distributed in space and time. **B.** There is a loss of individual muscle fibers in the myopathies. When motorneuron *a* fires, only fibers *1* and *3* remain. Therefore, the summated action potential, produced by adding individual action potentials from fibers *1* and *3,* is reduced in amplitude and duration. Although the motor unit territory has shrunk, the anterior horn cells are unaffected. As a result, a relatively normal number of these small, brief MUPs is produced. **C.** The neuropathies are characterized by involvement of most, if not all, of the peripheral axons. The terminal branches have been injured and the collateral to fiber *1* has been lost entirely. The summated action potential from fibers *2* through *5* is diminished in amplitude and duration. Depending on the severity of involvement, the motor unit territory may be diminished to a greater or lesser degree, and the number of MUPs correspondingly reduced. **D.** In the neuronopathies, the anterior horn cells are affected. As illustrated, motorneuron *b* has degenerated, leaving the muscle fibers formerly within its area without innervation. Anterior horn cell *a,* still intact, sends out additional terminal branches in an attempt to take over these fibers. In doing so, more muscle fibers become part of the motor unit subserved by Cell *a,* a total of seven instead of five fibers. These additional fibers add amplitude and duration to the summated action potential produced when Cell *a* fires (a so-called "giant" action potential). Although the territory controlled by the motor unit enlarges and the potentials are extremely large, the dropout of anterior horn cells leaves far fewer motorneurons to fire. As a result, the MUPs are reduced in number and even rare. (After *Norris FH: The EMG. A Guide and Atlas for Practical Electromyography. New York, Grune & Stratton, 1963, p 134).*

In diseases of the peripheral nerve, a number of alterations of the MUP may be evident, depending on the nature and severity of the condition. When a nerve has been severed completely, no voluntary MUPs will be seen. But if only some of the nerve fibers have been destroyed, the number of MUPs will be proportional to the number of remaining functional fibers.

One of the earliest signs of nerve regeneration and return of function is a significant increase in polyphasic potentials (so-called "nascent" MUPs). These may be large in amplitude and increased in duration, frequently firing at a slow rate. One or two such potentials are not an indication of complete return of function, however. In neuropathies related to systemic disorders, the number of MUPs usually is decreased, with an increase in polyphasic potentials commensurate with compensatory mechanisms of regeneration.

In myasthenia gravis, the affected muscles may show some variation in the amplitude of repetitively firing individual MUPs. On repeated effort, individual MUPs tend to decrease in amplitude and duration, perhaps indicative of "exhaustion" of the supply of neurotransmitter to some fibers in that motor unit. With a severe degree of junctional block, the number of MUPs decreases sharply.

Myopathic disorders, especially the dystrophies, produce marked changes in the MUP. The benign or slowly progressive myopathies with abnormal constituents

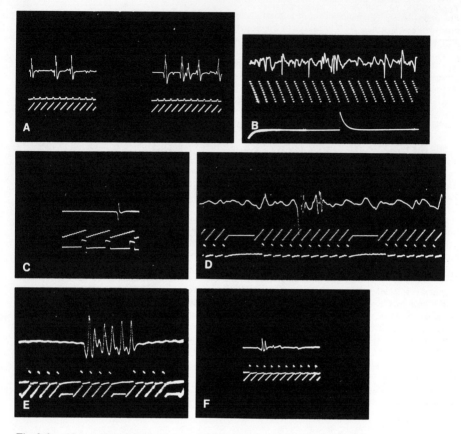

Fig. 3–9. Abnormal variations of normal potentials. **A.** "Giant" MUP, about 10 mV, recorded from a patient with amyotrophic lateral sclerosis from the abductor digiti quinti muscle. Monopolar needle electrode; minimum voluntary contraction; calibration, 1 mV, 10 msec/staircase. **B.** "Myopathic" MUP recorded from the deltoid muscle of a patient with polymyositis. Coaxial needle electrode; minimum voluntary contraction; calibration, 0.2 mV, 10 msec/staircase. **C.** Fasciculation recorded as in *A* from tibialis anterior; muscle at rest; Calibration, 1 mV, 1 msec/step. **D.** "Pony" ("satellite") potential following and locked to the polyphasic MUP. Recorded from the tibialis anterior; monopolar needle electrode; calibration, 1 mV, 1 msec/step. **E.** "Grouped" potential. This complex potential is better termed "grouped" than "polyphasic." Recorded from the first dorsal interosseus muscle, monopolar needle electrode; calibration, 1 mV, 1 msec/step. **F.** "Doublet" recorded from the gastrocnemius muscle, monopolar needle electrode. Calibration, 1 mV, 1 msec/step.

within the muscle (nemaline, sarcotubular, megaconical myopathies) show no, or relatively little, change in electrical characteristics.

In pseudohypertrophic muscular dystrophy, however, distinct alterations are noted. The MUPs are small in amplitude and of short duration (Fig. 3–9B). Over the loudspeaker, they emit a high-pitched sound. The interference pattern shows increased numbers of MUPs relative to the strength of contraction, and may be characterized by periodic waxing and waning of amplitude. The rate of firing is increased.

Table 3-2. METHOD OF GRADING THE SEVERITY OF FASCICULATIONS AND FIBRILLATIONS

Fasciculations or fibrillations (No. per minute)	Grade
1–2	1+
2–10	2+
10–30	3+
> 30 (continuous)	4+

In some myopathies, especially polymyositis, the incidence of polyphasic potentials is increased. The amplitude of the latter, in contrast to other polyphasic potentials, is small with a relatively short duration.

As the knowledge of the basic physiology of the motor unit advances and techniques of muscle histologic examination are improved, more information will be available for identification and differentiation of specific fiber-type disorders. Some reports of specific EMG findings in these conditions have been published (10) with correlation between histochemistry and ENM.

FASCICULATIONS   Fasciculation potentials result from spontaneous contractions of individual motor units (Fig. 3–9C). Their amplitude, duration, and waveform may vary but approximate those of MUPs. They occur in isolated fashion and must be differentiated from MUPs which result from minimal voluntary contraction. It therefore is important that the muscle be at rest in order to verify their presence. These potentials usually have a loud, "thump-like" sound, like typing on cardboard (Table 3–1). The needle may move or "jump" in synchrony with the electrical event.

The potentials are arhythmic and may be graded according to the frequency with which they occur (Table 3–2). If only one or two fasciculations are noted, they are described as 1+, 2 to 10 potentials over a period of 1 min are graded as 2+, with 3+ fasciculations equivalent to 10 or more/min. When continuous fasciculations are noted, they are graded as 4+. While these criteria are purely arbitrary, they provide a useful system of comparison. The size, duration, and shape of fasciculations resemble the MUPs in that particular disorder.

The origin of fasciculations is unknown. The term was coined by Denny–Brown and Pennybacker in 1938 (8) to distinguish these muscular twitches from fibrillations. They may persist after nerve block (13). They frequently are visible through the skin, especially in thin individuals. Trojaborg and Buchtal (20) noted that those occurring in motor neuron disease have a longer interval between successive discharges (about 3.5 sec or longer) than the "benign" fasciculations in normal muscle (about 0.8 sec). The other parameters of fasciculations—amplitude, duration, and shape—are similar in normal and diseased states.

Fasciculations are encountered most frequently in neuronopathies (motor neuron disease), especially the adult forms, but also are seen in some peripheral neuropathies, mostly in instances of nerve regeneration. They are considered pathological when associated with other abnormalities of MUPs and fibrillations. As an isolated finding, they are noted in normal individuals, especially in the lower extremities, about the eye, and small hand muscles. They are known to follow frequent vigorous exercise or injections of prostigmin.

MYOKYMIA   Myokymia is a synchronous discharge of several motor units. The electrical discharges appear as trains of MUPs from several units, lasting up to 0.5 sec (14). They have been reported in a variety of disorders, including multiple sclerosis and thyrotoxicosis, and as an isolated phenomenon.

TREMOR   Tremor, especially at rest, can be recorded by EMG. The EMG correlate of the clinical phenomenon consists of bursts of potentials, usually "distant" from the needle. Their parameters are those of MUPs with rhythmic discharge. The rhythm is related to the underlying disorder.

GROUPED DISCHARGES   MUP firing in groups of two or three potentials sometimes are noted. They may occur as spontaneous, irregular bursts (as fasciculations) or with a weak, sustained contraction. They are referred to as doublets or triplets. They have been reported to occur in normal muscles as well as in tetany, motor neuron disease, and parkinsonism (19) (Figs. 3–9E and 3–9F and Fig. 3–11D).

MUSCLE CRAMP   The EMG in muscle cramp displays a continuous discharge of MUPs at a high frequency for the duration of the cramp. A number of motor units are involved; thus a variety of sizes and shapes are seen to discharge recurrently. Muscle cramp is correlated with a variety of etiologies (17).

TETANY   The EMG in tetany shows bursts or continuous firing of MUPs similar to that seen in the interference pattern of normal voluntary contraction. Grouped discharges are seen in some muscles. They may be evoked by maneuvers used to elicit latent tetany (ischemia, direct percussion, etc.).

MYOTONIA   Clinically, myotonia consists of delayed relaxation following muscular contraction, either voluntary or evoked. The electrical discharges which accompany this phenomenon can be termed "myotonic discharges type I" (Fig. 3–10). All such discharges (both type I and type II, will be discussed later) have in common some anomaly of the muscle membrane that leads to repetitive discharge, i.e., autorhythmicity of firing.

Such discharges can be detected and displayed by EMG. They have been described as "dive bomber" potentials because their sound is similar to that of an airplane in a dive. On the oscilloscope, they appear as repetitive MUPs which occur in trains with progressive decrement of amplitude and increase of interval between potentials. These phenomena account for the falloff in volume and pitch, respectively (4). Such discharges are found in cases of myotonia congenita, myotonic dystrophy, polymyositis, the hyperkalemic form of periodic paralysis, and the myopathy of acid maltase deficiency. They are evoked by voluntary contraction, percussion of the muscle, and movement of the needle electrode (Table 3–3).

Spontaneous trains of potentials which resemble type I myotonic discharges because they are repetitive and self-sustaining can be seen in a number of conditions in the *absence* of clinical myotonia (Fig. 3–10). The nomenclature of this category is confusing. The use of the suffix "myotonia" (e.g., "electromyographic myotonia," "pseudomyotonia," "denervation myotonia," or "subclinical myotonia") implies a relationship to the clinical phenomenon which may or may not be real.

Moreover, these discharges differ from those which accompany clinical myotonia in that they are usually nondecremental, i.e., show the same amplitude for

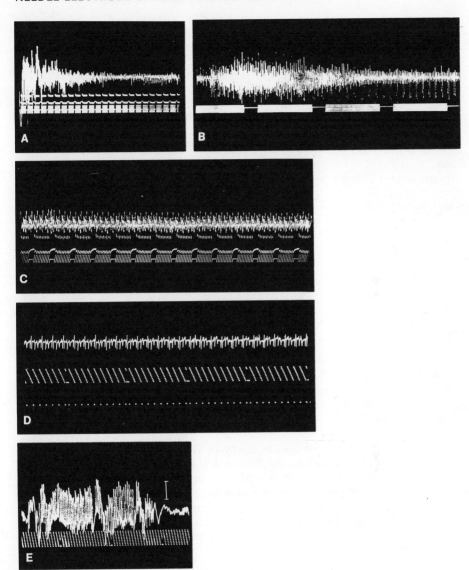

Fig. 3–10. Myotonic discharges. **A.** Type I myotonic discharge recorded from the tibialis posterior from a patient with myotonic dystrophy, coaxial needle electrode recording. Myotonic discharge evoked by needle insertion. Calibration, 1 mV, 100 msec. **B.** Type I myotonic discharge recorded from the opponens pollicis muscle from a patient with myotonic dystrophy, coaxial needle electrode recording. Calibration, as in *A*, 1 sec/solid time marker. **C.** Type II myotonic discharge recorded from the left biceps brachii, coaxial needle recording. Calibration, 100 µV, 10 msec/staircase. **D.** Same as *C* later on in the discharge. Note the lack of decrescendo pattern and the complex or grouped potentials in *C* and *D* (in contrast to *A* and *B*). Time, 10 msec/staircase. **E.** Type II myotonic discharge (bizarre high-frequency potentials) from a patient with motor neuron disease. First dorsal interosseus muscle. Calibration, 100 µV, 10 msec/staircase.

Table 3-3. MYOTONIC DISCHARGES

	Type I	Type II
Clinical Myotonia	present	absent
Clinical Correlation	Myotonia Congenita	Denervation
	Myotonic Dystrophy	Anterior horn cell
	Polymyositis	Root Syndromes
	Hyperkalemic PP	Acquired myopathies
	Acid Maltase def.	
Evoked by voluntary contraction, percussion of muscle and needle insertion	Yes	Yes
Decrescendo Pattern (dive-bomber)	Yes	Usually no
MUP within the train		
Duration	Relatively normal	Short
Amplitude	Relatively normal	Low
Wave form	Relatively normal	Polyphasic
Duration of train	3–10 sec	1) very brief, e.g., 1 sec.—"bizarre high-frequency potentials" or 2) sustained, up to several minutes.

the duration of the discharge. The potentials within the train are usually smaller in amplitude (<0.5 mV) and duration (<5 msec) and are more polyphasic or "grouped" than those seen in the trains of dive-bomber potentials which accompany clinical myotonia (Table 3–3). They may be brief (termed "bizarre high-frequency potentials" by some), or quite prolonged, even several minutes in duration.

This type of discharge has been termed type II to distinguish it from the decremental, shorter trains which accompany clinical myotonia, type I (4). The mechanism of such discharges is unknown but may be related (as are type I myotonic discharges) to an abnormality of the muscle membrane which gives rise to an unstable resting membrane potential. Type II myotonic discharges can be seen in a variety of disorders which affect the lower motor neuron and muscle, including diseases of the spinal roots and anterior horn cells (3), and the acquired myopathies.

Potentials Not Encountered in Most Normal States

FIBRILLATIONS Unlike fasciculations, which may be seen through the intact skin and commonly are present in normal persons, fibrillations are visible only by direct, careful inspection of the bared muscle surface in a good light as minute, brief movements. Furthermore, they rarely occur in normal individuals, except for one or two occasional discharges. These potentials are of short duration (1–2 msec), low amplitude (10–50 μV), and have a characteristic "crackling" sound rather like wrinkling cellophane. They are bi- or triphasic, have an initial positive spike, may occur at regular (rare) or irregular intervals, and can be provoked by movement of the needle electrode, or by tapping or squeezing the muscle.

Fibrillations may occur with the muscle at rest, or after passive movements or voluntary contraction. They may be graded according to the number observed per

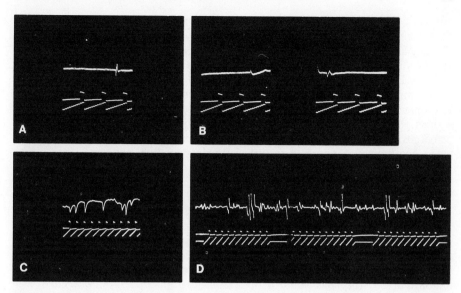

Fig. 3–11. Potentials not encountered in most normal states. **A.** Fibrillation potential recorded from the gastrocnemius muscle of a patient with amyotrophic lateral sclerosis, monopolar needle recording. Calibration, 100 μV. **B.** Same as *A,* except recording taken from the left abductor digiti quinti. Calibration, 100 μV. **C.** Positive sharp waves recorded from the left extensor digitorum brevis, monopolar needle electrode recording. Calibration, 100 μV. **D.** Doublets and triplets recorded from the right gastrocnemius muscle, coaxial needle electrode. Calibration, 1 μV.

unit time (1 to 4+) in a manner analogous to fasciculations (Table 3–2). They should be searched for not only at rest, but after needle movement and voluntary contraction (Fig. 3–11 A and B).

Fibrillation potentials are encountered in instances of denervation and thus commonly are referred to as "denervation potentials." This may be a misnomer, because they have been described in conditions not presently considered primary neurogenic. They occur, however, in greatest numbers in severe nerve lesions. They also are present in anterior horn cell disease and even in the myopathies, especially polymyositis. The presence of fibrillations without additional information does not indicate the site of the lesion. They are difficult to distinguish from the small, sharp MUPs found in some myopathies.

As with fasciculations and other discharges, the origin and pathogenesis of fibrillations is not clear. They have been considered to be discharges from single muscle fibers, but proof of their origin and the generation of the spike is not established. After poliomyelitis, they may persist in affected muscles for many years. They are not a prominent feature of the infantile form of motor neuron disease, but are seen in scattered fashion in the adult forms. In neuropathies, the general rule is that the more acute the process, the more prominent the fibrillations.

With reinnervation, fibrillatory activity tends to subside. It usually is not present in upper motor neuron lesions, although occasional fibrillations may be seen. Whether this is the result of transneuronal degeneration or a secondary phenomenon of nerve compression is not clear. Fibrillations are not seen in atrophy of muscle secondary to disuse.

POSITIVE WAVES   Positive waves consist of a single-phase positive discharge. They are usually 2–10 msec in duration and vary in amplitude from 20 to 300 μ V. They are encountered in the same conditions, and their frequency and pattern of occurrance are the same, as fibrillations. Like the latter, their origin is unclear, but may be related to irritation of single injured muscle fibers (Fig. 3–11C).

In summary, with needle electrode studies, a careful examination must include 1) proper choice of muscles to be examined, 2) observation of discharges under various physiologic states of the muscle, 3) identification of variations of normal potentials, 4) search for abnormal potentials, 5) quantitative analysis of the potentials when indicated, and 6) a record of the data for final analysis.

MOTOR UNIT TERRITORY STUDIES

The spike of the MUP arises from many muscle fibers which summate more-or-less synchronously even though separated by some distance. An estimate of the size of the motor unit (i.e., the territory or area subtended by the muscle fibers belonging to that motor unit) cannot be made with a single needle electrode. The study of motor unit territory has value in neuromuscular disorders. Values have been obtained for a number of conditions (5, 12). In amyotrophic lateral sclerosis, for example, there is an increase in the size of the motor unit territory. It tends to decrease in severe myopathies. The technique has value in instances where other studies fail to define the site of pathology.

To measure motor unit territory, a multielectrode needle (Ch. 1, Fig. 1–2A) is employed. This multiaxial needle is inserted into a muscle and adjusted in depth so that the maximal discharge of a single MUP is near the center electrodes. Serial or simultaneous recordings are made from each electrode. The distance between each of the electrode tips, the amplitude of each of the recorded potentials, and their differences as to time of discharge are used to calculate the territory size. Another technique has been described by Norris (18).

PARAMETERS OF THE DISCHARGES

The parameters of the electrical discharges discussed in this chapter are summarized in Table 3–1. Minor differences may be noted from values quoted by other authors; these may be related to equipment differences.

PATHOPHYSIOLOGY OF ELECTROMYOGRAPHY

The EMG procedures described in this chapter are applicable to the majority of neuromuscular diseases. When the findings are correlated with other ENM parameters, they play a major role in diagnosis. A comprehensive correlation of all ENM studies will be found in Chapter 5, Table 5–1.

Functional Disorders and Upper Motor Neuron Diseases

In hysteria and malingering, the various EMG parameters are normal. The rate of MUP firing is irregular and bizarre patterns of voluntary MUPs are common, but they are commensurate with the mechanical contraction. Furthermore, using two channels for EMG recording—one from agonist and another from antagonist —one often can demonstrate a normal interference pattern in an allegedly paretic muscle (e.g., Hoover's sign). Provided adequate sampling is obtained, negative results have important diagnostic and medicolegal implications.

In upper motor neuron lesions, the total number of MUPs is reduced proportional to the strength of contraction. The rate of firing likewise is decreased and there occasionally is a slight increase in the number of polyphasic MUPs. In uncomplicated upper motor neuron lesions, the remainder of the EMG is within normal limits.

Anterior Horn Cell Diseases

In the neuronopathies such as poliomyelitis and amyotrophic lateral sclerosis, insertion activity is increased. Fibrillations and positive waves are seen following insertion of the needle but often occur spontaneously, and numerous fasciculations frequently are present. Although fasciculations can be seen in normal individuals and also in diseases other than anterior horn cell involvement, they are typical of the latter.

On voluntary contraction, the MUPs are increased in amplitude and duration. These so called "giant" MUPs result from enlargement of the motor unit territory (terminal collateral sprouting of the motor nerve). There is a decrease in the total number of MUPs; thus the interference pattern is reduced and discrete MUPs often are seen with maximal voluntary effort. Consistent with the process of denervation–reinnervation, there is an increase in polyphasic MUPs which are frequently of large amplitude and long duration. The rate of firing of the MUPs, especially the "giants," usually is decreased. Type II myotonic discharges rarely are observed.

Neuropathies

While various neuropathies show similar qualitative EMG changes, they differ considerably in degree depending on the location and nature of the pathology.

In complete nerve transection, voluntary motor units are absent from the onset; the insertion potentials initially are decreased to absent and, after 7–21 days, there is increased irritability. Many fibrillations and positive waves are present in the denervated muscles. If no recovery takes place in the transected nerve and there is total atrophy of the involved muscles, electrical silence is the rule. With recovery, the fibrillations and positive waves gradually subside. Polyphasic potentials are present in the early recovery phase. Few in number at first, they increase with reinnervation and subside to a near normal percentage of potentials with complete recovery. Individual motor units, firing slowly and irregularly, gradually intermix with and replace the polyphasic units.

With multiple-root involvement as in the Guillain–Barré syndrome, the location and degree of denervation is consistent with the site and severity of the pathology. With moderate to severe involvement, the MUPs are reduced in number and their rate of firing decreased. With recovery, polyphasic potentials frequently precede development of normal MUPs. The latter are large in amplitude and long in duration. Fasciculations occur infrequently during recovery.

In polyneuropathy associated with chronic disorders such as diabetes, the EMG changes may be more subtle. The amount of denervation is usually moderate to minimal. Fibrillations and positive waves frequently can be evoked on needle movement, but are not abundant spontaneously. Fasciculations may be present, but are infrequent. The amplitude and duration of MUPs are usually normal, but the total number may be reduced slightly with a normal complement relative to the strength of contraction. It is common to find an increased number of polyphasic potentials.

Single-root lesions, such as a herniated nucleus pulposus compressing the motor fibers, will produce changes in those muscles supplied by that root, including those of the posterior primary rami. Individual peripheral nerve lesions will produce similar findings in the muscles innervated by that nerve. With the knowledge of segmental and peripheral nerve innervation, the site of involvement, i.e., nerve root or peripheral nerve, can be determined. With multiple sites of involvement, e.g., nerve root lesion with diabetic neuropathy, an overlapping pattern of abnormality occasionally is produced.

Disorders of the Myoneural Junction

In myoneural junction disorders, the insertion potentials are normal; no denervation potentials or fasciculations are present. On sustained weak contraction, the amplitude of an individual MUP may be seen to vary. With repeated maximal contraction of affected muscles, the rate of firing tends to decline, and the amplitude and duration of individual MUPs diminishes. The number of polyphasic potentials is normal.

Myopathies

The nature of the myopathic disturbance determines to some degree the pattern of EMG abnormaly.

In progressive muscular dystrophy, insertion activity is normal or slightly increased. Usually no denervation potentials are present; no fasciculations are observed. The MUPs are of low amplitude and short duration, and are increased in number relative to the strength of contraction ("myopathic MUPs"). The rate of firing is rapid and, in advanced disease, the total number of MUPs is decreased. The short duration and low amplitude of the MUPs are related to a decrease in the size of motor unit territory. There is an increase in number of polyphasic potentials, which are also of low amplitude.

Inflammatory myopathies, especially in the acute phase, show conspicuous abnormalities. There is increased irritability on insertion. Fibrillations and positive waves often are present and are difficult to distinguish from the myopathic MUPs. Short-duration, low-amplitude polyphasic potentials are increased in number. The myopathic potentials may be interlaced with normal MUPs, consistent with the pathology of diseased as well as normal fibers seen on muscle biopsy. Types I and II myotonic discharges may be present in inflammatory myopathies.

SUMMARY OF STEPS IN PERFORMING ELECTROMYOGRAPHY (NEEDLE ELECTRODE STUDIES)

Step 1. As with NSS, (a) familiarize yourself with the patient's history and physical examination reports; (b) introduce yourself to the patient and proceed with any necessary history and neurologic examination, with special attention to the sensory and motor systems. The examiner should perform one or two needle electrode studies on himself to gain first-hand experience with the sensation and the procedure.

Step 2. Turn on the power for the equipment and check the dial settings: a) VERTICAL POSITION of the trace; b) FOCUS; c) TRACE INTENSITY; d) SWEEP SPEED: Initially set the oscilloscope sweep speed at 10 msec/cm. Occasionally other sweep speeds will be needed in order to gauge the duration of MUPs more accurately. At faster sweep speeds, potentials may appear double or triple due to rapid recurrent trace sweep, making them difficult to interpret visually; (e) CALIBRATION SETTINGS: Initially set the calibration at 50 or 100 μV. The height of larger potentials is measured more easily at calibration settings of 1–5 mV; f) when using a calibration signal on a second channel, be certain both gain settings are the same; and g) set the SELECTOR dial for EMG.

Step 3. Select an EMG needle. Use a 1½-in. needle for obese individuals or when deep muscles are to be examined; and a ¾-in. needle for children or lean individuals. Verify that the needle has been sterilized properly. Impedence should be checked periodically. If a monopolar needle is being used, place the indifferent electrode on the skin in proximity to the needle over the muscle being tested.

Step 4. Plug the wires from the needle electrode into the machine outlet, along with the ground wire.

Step 5. Cleanse the skin with alcohol over the test area. This is done each time the needle is inserted.

Step 6. Obtain muscle relaxation and be prepared to listen to the sound of insertion activity. Let the patient know when you are about to proceed.

Step 7. Be certain you are testing the correct muscle by its location on the basis of surface anatomy and also by its function. Insert the needle into the muscle in a swift, smooth movement and listen to the insertion potentials and any potentials that follow. Normally there will be a brief burst of insertion activity followed by silence.

Step 8. Allow the needle electrode to remain in position and look–listen for any abnormalities. Wait about 15–30 sec; if no abnormalities are noted, then proceed with the next step. If any abnormalities are noted, investigate the area further.

a. If fasciculations are present, allow the needle to remain in place and note the number/unit time as well as amplitude and waveform.

b. If fibrillations or positive waves are noted after insertion activity, then record how long they persist, together with their size and frequency. If they do not occur spontaneously or on insertion, see if they can be evoked by tapping or squeezing the muscle near the needle.

Step 9. Have the patient produce a minimal contraction to study individual MUPs. Record a) amplitude, b) duration, c) frequency of discharge, d) approximate number of polyphasic potentials in relation to the total number of MUPs, and e) the number of MUPs relative to varying strengths of contraction. Reduce the gain when necessary and/or alter the time scale to obtain an estimate of the size and duration of the individual potentials. If necessary, make a permanent record to analyze for the percentage of polyphasic potentials.

Step 10. Have the patient contract the muscle maximally and note the interference pattern, that is, how many MUPs fill the oscilloscope screen.

Step 11. Note what happens when the patient is asked to relax. Do the potentials cease abruptly, as usually occurs in normal individuals, or does relaxation occur gradually, as in myotonia with the characteristic type I discharge?

Step 12. If the patient cannot contract the muscle voluntarily, note what happens if the muscle is lengthened passively and released by moving the appropriate joint briskly.

Step 13. Sample several areas of the muscle, using the "quadrant" technique, then proceed to the next muscle to be tested. Record the findings for that muscle before proceeding to the next.

Step 14. Continue to test all necessary muscles until you are satisfied that maximum information has been obtained. If the patient seems to be fatigued, or if the test is unusually long, ask the patient to return on another day for further studies.

Step 15. After concluding the procedure, wipe the needle gently and place it in an appropriate container for sterilization. Disconnect all wires from the patient. Check for areas of active bleeding from the punctures. After completing all studies and *before* the patient is dismissed, the electroneuromyographer should have a clear concept of the site, degree, and, if possible, the nature of the problem.

USE OF THE TAPE RECORDER

Although a tape recorder (Fig. 3–12) is not essential for EMG, it is most valuable for maintaining a permanent file and for teaching. It may be used to transmit information concerning a specific patient to another electroneuromyographer or for computer analysis of data. The examiner should be familiar with the recorder controls. He should try the unit prior to use with patients.

The speed should be set at 7½ in./sec because this gives the best fidelity and the least distortion on playback. A microphone is supplied with the unit so that the recording may be labeled vocally on a second channel throughout the testing procedure. In some units, when the microphone switch is left at ON, the EMG amplifier is inoperable for EMG or for playback from the tape; this switch should be turned to OFF when the microphone is not in use. Also, the EMG amplifiers may be bypassed if the recorder is left on PLAYBACK; thus, the oscilloscope display and the audio system will not function in this position. Consult the operations manual for the details of the specific unit available to you.

Summary of Steps in Using the Tape Recorder

Step 1. Prepare tape recorder for use: a) thread tape through recording head as per directions; b) turn power on; c) set recording speed at 7½ in./sec; d) plug microphone into labeled jack box on the machine; e) turn microphone switch to ON; and f) activate RECORD switch with START.

Step 2. Be certain that the needle electrode has been inserted in the area for recording.

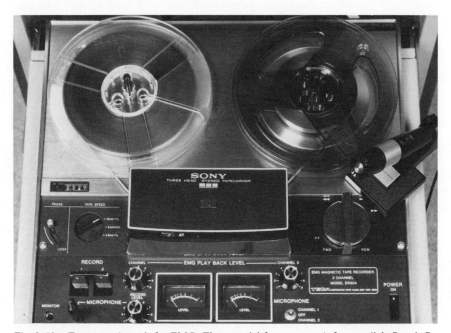

Fig. 3–12. Tape recorder unit for EMG. The essential features are *A,* footage dial; *B* and *C,* volume control for channels *1* and *2,* respectively; *D* and *E,* volt meters to monitor channels *1* and *2,* respectively; *F,* volume control for the microphone; *G,* selector switch for channels *1* and *2;* and *H,* microphone.

Table 3-4. EXAMPLE OF PATIENT TAPE RECORD

Date	Patient	Tape Box No.	Footage	Diagnosis	Remarks
1/1/75	Smith, J.	3	0000–0051	Carpal Tunnel Syndrome	Fibrillation in right abductor pollicis brevis
1/2/75	Jones, M.	3	0055–0095	Myotonic Dystrophy	Myotonic discharges

Step 3. Over the microphone identify: a) examiner's name; b) date and time; c) patient's name and identifying number; d) the muscle being tested; e) the calibration setting, sweep speed, and type of needle used; and f) any additional information for teaching such as the provisional diagnosis. Then turn the microphone to OFF and continue to record. Record a calibration signal and time base on one channel of the tape.

Step 4. Allow the tape to run and record the appropriate discharges. If sensitivity or sweep speed is altered, be certain to note this over the microphone and place a new calibration signal on the tape. When the recording is finished, stop the recorder. It is advisable to play back a portion of the record to be certain that you have recorded correctly.

Step 5. Most tape recorders have a footage dial which indicates the place on the tape at which each given event has been recorded. Number each tape (on the tape box) and keep a notebook record with the tape number, the patient, the date, the diagnosis, etc., for reference (Table 3–4). Record the footage-dial setting for each patient on the tape box and also in the notebook. Be certain to leave the tape at the last footage dial number recorded in the book when you are listening to a replay; otherwise you or someone else may erase important data.

ARTIFACTS AND SOURCES OF ERROR (see also Chapter 2)

There are certain characteristic sights and sounds which are recognizable as artifacts. The beginner should produce these on purpose in order to recognize them easily.

60-Hz Interference

60 Hz interference is by far the most common artifact. It is readily recognized on the oscilloscope by its highly regular discharge in the 60 Hz frequency (Ch. 2, Fig. 2–21). When the sensitivity (gain control) is high, as is necessary for needle electrode studies, 60 Hz interference can be detected if the equipment is not grounded properly, if the patient is not grounded, or if the patient or examiner is in a position to conduct such interference to the equipment. The ground wire to the equipment or the patient may be broken along its course, or a needle or its wire to the plug may break due to improper handling and care. When this artifact is present, check grounds first then look for loose connections or completely or partially broken electrode wires. It may be necessary to change one lead at a time to detect the faulty one. A volt-ohmmeter may be used to advantage to detect breaks in the circuitry.

Audio Feedback

In some equipment, the "feedback phenomenon" of the audio amplifiers also may appear as a confusing artifact (Ch. 2, Fig. 2–21). It may be due to reverberation from the audio system. It can be eliminated by reducing the volume or separating

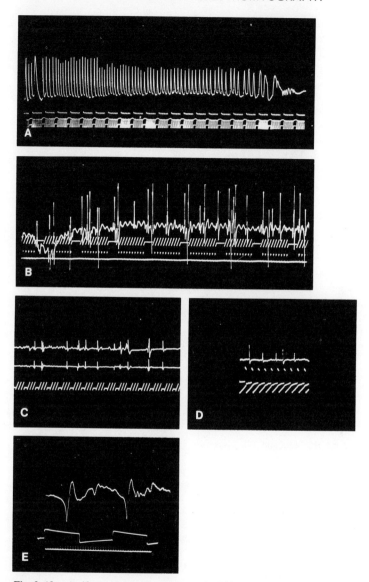

Fig. 3–13. Artifacts and sources of error. **A.** This artifact was produced when the wire from a needle electrode was broken. **B.** 60–cycle interference. The sinusoidal distortion of the base line was produced by a loose ground electrode. Recording with monopolar needle electrodes from the tibialis anterior muscle. **C.** This recording illustrates the effect of a defective needle electrode. The top tracing represents a new needle; the bottom tracing, a needle with a blistered Teflon coating. Recording from the tibialis anterior muscle, monopolar needle electrodes. **D.** Nerve potentials recorded from the left tibialis posterior, monopolar needle electrode. Calibration, 100 μV.
E. Irregular artifact caused by bumping the needle. Occasionally a similar artifact can be produced by bumping the table or other electrical connections.

the loudspeaker system from the remainder of the equipment. High-frequency feedback also may be caused by poor connections between the audio amplifiers and the needle electrodes.

Movement

Tapping the patient or stamping one's foot on the floor may produce a brief interruption of the trace, and a "thump" will be heard. Bumping into the wires from the needle electrodes, scratching or touching the patient all may produce confusing artifacts (Fig. 3–3A).

Miscellaneous

The Teflon insulation on monopolar needles requires careful handling. It can be scraped off accidently or dissolved by certain solutions (e.g., Zephiran and gas autoclaving) (Ch. 1, Fig. 1–3). Loss of part of the coating of a monopolar electrode may alter the parameters of the recorded potentials (Fig. 3–13B). When a monopolar needle electrode is inserted into a partially denervated muscle and the indifferent electrode is placed over an adjacent, healthy muscle, the latter will pick up distant motor units with normal parameters. Therefore, when monopolar needles are used, it is important to place the indifferent electrode *over* the muscle being tested. Other artifacts include a loose wire (Fig. 3–13C), nerve potentials (Fig. 3–13D), and movement of equipment (Fig. 3–13E).

REFERENCES

1. Adrian ED, Bronck DW: The discharge of impulses in motor nerve fibers. J Physiol (Lond) 67: 119–151, 1929
1a. Basmajian JB, Clifford HC, McLeod WD, Nunnally HN: Computors in Electromyography. Reading, Mass, Butterworth, 1975, p 126
2. Brandstater ME, Lambert EH: Motor unit anatomy: type and special arrangement of muscle fibers. In Desmedt JE (ed): New Developments in Electromyography and Clinical Neurophysiology, Vol I. Basel, Karger, 1973, pp 14–22
3. Brumlik J, Cuetter AC: Denervation myotonia: a subclinical electromyographic finding. Electromyography 9: 297–310, 1969
4. Brumlik J, Drechsler B, Vannin TM: The myotonic discharge in various neurological syndromes: a neurophysiological analysis. Electromyography 10: 369–383, 1970
5. Buchtal F, Rosenfalck P, Erminio F: Motor unit territory and fiber density in myopathies. Neurology (Minneap) 10: 398, 1960
6. Chantraine A: EMG examination of the anal and urethral sphincters. In Desmedt JE(ed): New Developments in Electromyography and Clinical Neurophysiology, Vol II. Basel, Karger, 1973, pp 421–432
6a. Delagi EF, Perotto A: Clinical Electromyography of the Hand. Arch Phys Med Rehabil 57: 66–69, 1976
7. Denny–Brown D: Interpretation of the electromyogram. Arch Neurol 61: 99, 1949
8. Denny–Brown D, Pennypacker JB: Fibrillation and fasciculation in voluntary muscle. Brain 61: 311–344, 1938
9. Ekstedt J: Human single muscle fiber action potentials. Acta Physiol Scand [Suppl] 226 (61): 1–96, 1964
10. Engel WK: Classification of neuromuscular disorders. Biol Birth Defects: Original article series 2: 218–237, 1971

11. Engel WK, Warmolts JR: The motor unit. In Desmedt JE (ed): New Developments in Electromyography and Clinical Neurophysiology, Vol I. Basel, Karger, 1973, 141–177
12. Erminio F, Buchtal F, Rosenfalck P: Motor unit territory and muscle fiber concentration in paresis due to peripheral nerve injury and anterior horn cell involvement. Neurology (Minneap) 9: 657, 1959
13. Forster FM, Alpers BJ: Site of origin of fasciculations in voluntary muscle. Arch Neurol Psychiatry (Chicago) 51: 264, 1944
14. Gardner–Medwin D, Walton JN: Myokymia with impaired muscular relaxation. Lancet 1: 127–130, 1969
15. Granit R: The Basis of Motor Control. New York, Academic Press, 1970, p 346
16. Lambert EH: Electromyography in amyotrophic lateral sclerosis. In Norris F, Kurland L (eds): Motor Neuron Diseases. New York, Grune & Stratton, 1969, p 138
17. Layzer RB, Rowland FP: The etiology of muscle cramps. N Engl J Med 285: 31–41, 1971
18. Norris FH: The EMG. A Guide and Atlas for Practical Electromyography. New York, Grune & Stratton, 1963, p 134
19. Simpson JA (ed): (Part B) Neuromuscular Diseases. In Buchtal F (ed): Electromyography, Vol 16. In Remond A (ed): Handbook of Electroencephalography and Clinical Neurophysiology. Amsterdam, Elsevier, 1973, p 162
20. Trojaborg W, Buchtal F: Malignant and benign fasciculations. Acta Neurol Scand [Suppl] 41(13): 251–254, 1965
21. Weddel G, Feinstein B, Pattle RE: The electrical activity of voluntary muscle in man under normal and pathological conditions. Brain 67: 178–257, 1944

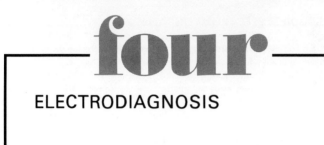

ELECTRODIAGNOSIS

Electrodiagnosis may be defined as the application of electric current to nerve and muscle to determine clinical function. Although the techniques germane to EMG and NCV studies have received greater attention, EDX is the parent technique. For a more complete account of the history and apparatus used in electrodiagnosis, the reader is referred to Licht. (1)

Over the years, dating back to the 1800s, various parameters of study have been developed, including stimulation with faradic and galvanic current, rheobase, chronaxie, strength-duration curve, galvanic tetanus ratio, and repetitive stimulus curve. Before these parameters are discussed, the technique of examination will be described.

TECHNIQUE OF EXAMINATION

General

A principle in EDX is the determination of the least amount of stimulus required to produce a minimum twitch in a muscle. Because this twitch in a normal muscle may be obtained most easily by stimulation at the point where the main nerve trunk enters the muscle (the motor point), this must be located first. Every EDX laboratory should have available anatomic charts showing the motor points of various muscles on a surface diagram of the body. This approximate location, however, must be verified by exploration with a stimulating electrode in order to locate that point at which the smallest twitch is produced by the least current. At times, especially in advanced denervation, the amount of current needed to produce the smallest twitch will be great. Therefore, it usually is advisable to test a homologous normal muscle first to determine the motor point and the approximate amount of current needed. The diseased muscle then may be studied with greater confidence. Further, the muscle may become irritable in denervation, causing the motor point to lose its specificity and the area from which minimal twitch may be elicited to enlarge. In this instance, the motor point is "easier to find."

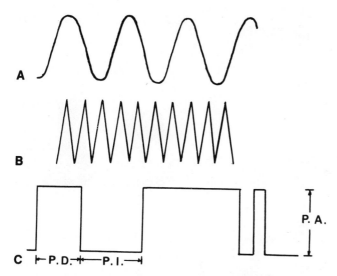

Fig. 4–1. Square-wave stimuli delivered by the EDX unit compared with other wave forms.
A. Sixty-cycle alternating current (commercial type, not used for biologic stimulation studies).
B. Faradic current produced by faradic coil; rapid "make" and "break" of coil produces pulses of
approximately 1 msec each. **C.** Square-wave pulses: P.A., pulse amplitude; P.D., pulse duration;
P.I., pulse interval.

Equipment

Before conducting any EDX study, familiarity with the equipment is essential (Fig. 4–3).

Standard EDX equipment consists of three units:

1. An amperage control and milliammeter from which the delivered current can be read. Because skin resistance is variable, constant-current stimulators are essential. If a constant-voltage stimulator were used, variable skin resistance might permit excess current to enter the tissue. Because it is current and not voltage that stimulates, the response would not be constant. The constant-current stimulator is designed to compensate for variable skin resistance, and alters the voltage output accordingly.

2. One or more controls to govern impulse duration.

3. One or more controls to vary impulse interval.

The EDX apparatus delivers square-wave impulses. By means of these controls, the examiner is able to vary the amplitude (current), interval (length of time between pulses) and duration of the impulse (Fig. 4–1).

Two electrodes are used, one stimulating and the other indifferent. A switch controls the polarity of the two electrodes, so that either can be made anode or cathode. The stimulating electrode may be of various shapes and sizes, but usually consists of a ball electrode measuring 1 or 2 cm. in spherical diameter, covered with felt. The indifferent electrode is a piece of clothcovered wire mesh measuring several square inches in area (Fig. 1–2). Both electrodes are thoroughly soaked in saline to provide good skin contact. Electrode jelly is rarely necessary. Care must

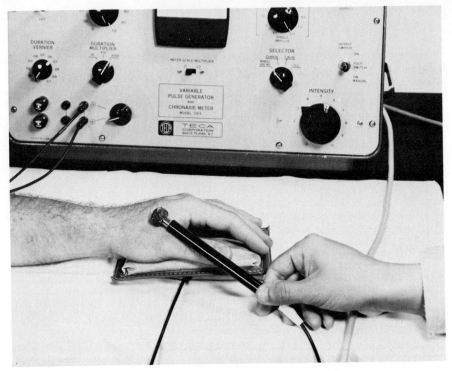

Fig. 4–2. Patient positioned for EDX study of left first dorsal interosseous muscle. Patient's hand rests on indifferent electrode (or anode); examiner holds the stimulating electrode over motor point of muscle. Stimuli are delivered by means of foot–pedal switch (on floor, not shown) so that examiner can operate equipment controls with his other hand.

be taken to prevent the electrodes from drying out during the test. If the electrodes do dry out, the amount of voltage required to produce minimal twitch becomes large; most likely no visible twitch will occur even with large amounts of current.

Position of the Patient

In performing the test, the subject must be at complete rest. He may either lie on a cart or, if only one or two muscles are to be tested and they are easily accessible, he may sit with the limb to be tested supported on a suitable table. He should not touch grounded metal objects.

The Motor Point

Once the patient has been properly positioned (Fig. 4–2), the indifferent electrode is placed in contact with the skin of the same extremity. The examiner should avoid placing the indifferent electrode on a limb other than the one tested to prevent electrical current from being conducted to other parts of the body. Although ordinary light will suffice, it is often desirable to obtain a source of oblique lighting across the muscle, such as a floor lamp with a reflector.

In order to determine the motor point, it is appropriate to use a current pulse of long duration, such as 300 msec (note that all time units in EDX are in milliseconds). The pulse interval is immaterial; 1,000 msec can be used as the pulse interval, or single pulses can be delivered at the examiner's discretion. The stimulating electrode (cathode) is applied to the skin approximately at the motor point, and a stimulus is given. The stimulus never is turned on before the stimulating electrode is in contact with the skin; similarly, the current is always switched off before the electrode is removed. If this is not done, unpleasant shocks may occur.

At the onset, the milliammeter should read 1 ma. Single pulses are delivered to the muscle either by means of the switch on the control panel or by the foot-pedal switch (Fig. 4–3). The current then can be increased with reasonable rapidity, ½ ma. at a time, until a minimum twitch is observed. In order to determine whether less current will produce a minimum twitch, the examiner then moves the electrode in every direction, lowering the amount of current as the electrode is moved. When

Fig. 4–3. Identification of the three main components of the EDX unit. **A.** Polarity control for stimulating electrodes. **B.** Input jacks for stimulating electrodes. **C.** Duration vernier control for *E.* **D.** Duration multiplier control for *E.* **E.** Pulse duration control. **F.** Meter scale multiplier. **G.** Miliammeter. **H.** Pulse interval control. **I.** Output switch for manual or foot–switch operation. **J.** Selector control for rheobase, chronaxie, and galvanic (D.C.) current. **K.** Intensity (amperage) control for pulse amplitude. **L.** Connecting wire to foot–pedal switch.

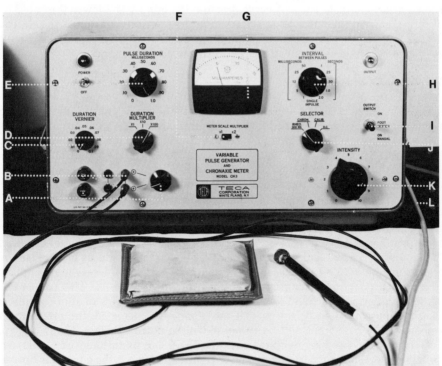

Table 4-1. ELECTRODIAGNOSTIC STUDIES

Parameter	Normal	Denervation
Faradic-galvanic*	F+, G+	F−, G+
Rheobase ratio	Over 1.5	Less than 1.0
Rheobase	5–8 ma	Less than 3 ma.
Chronaxie	Less than 1 msec.	More than 1.0 msec
S–D curve	Nerve	Muscle, with discontinuities
GTR	Over 3.0	Less than 3.0; approx. 1.0
R–S (S–I) curve	Straight	Ascending

*+ =response present; − =response absent.

the point of response to minimum stimulus is found, the motor point has been located. The location is marked on the skin with a suitable device. The electrode is not moved from this point during any subsequent procedures.

PARAMETERS: NORMAL AND ABNORMAL

Clinical applications of EDX techniques are based on the fact that a nerve-muscle preparation is differentially sensitive to currents of long and short duration. Assuming a constant stimulus strength, muscle is relatively insensitive to currents of very brief duration; conversely, nerve is quite sensitive to currents of this character. When a muscle's nerve supply is intact, the parameters (such as chronaxie) assume the electrical characteristics of nerve, because the latter has a lower threshold to electrical current than muscle. In denervation the preparation assumes the electrical characteristics of muscle alone. If a muscle is partly denervated or partly reinnervated, the responses will fall between these two extremes.

Faradic and Galvanic Current

The earliest clinical studies utilized galvanic and faradic current. It was found that if sufficient current were allowed to flow, galvanic current (i.e., that produced from an ordinary battery) would cause a muscle to twitch when the switch was opened and closed. This response occurs only during the opening (break) and closing (make) of the circuit, not while the current flows. However, a muscle does not need a nerve supply in order to respond to such galvanic current; therefore, this response only demonstrates the presence of functioning muscle. The absence of a response to galvanic current is known as the "cadaveric" response and is present only in complete atrophy and the paralytic stage of periodic paralysis. Faradic current, on the other hand, consists of a series of rapid pulses produced by the so-called "inductorium." The rapid make and break of the circuit produces brief pulses of approximately 1/750–1/1,000 sec. When pulses of such brief duration are applied to a normal neuromuscular preparation, contraction will result. This occurs because the nerve is intact and has a lower threshold to currents of short duration than the muscle "alone." However, if the muscle is denervated, the preparation responds as muscle alone and no response will be noted (Table 4–1).

Galvanic response may be tested with the EDX unit by turning the SELECTOR switch to D.C. This will permit galvanic current to flow when the current is turned on by means of the OUTPUT (stimulus) SWITCH (Fig. 4–3). The current is increased by means of the INTENSITY control as described earlier. Because the exact number of milliamperes is not specified in this test, the responses are recorded as either "present" or "absent." This lack of quantification detracts from the usefulness of the test, because there obviously is some difference between a muscle which responds to low amounts of direct current and a muscle which requires much more. To stimulate with faradic current, the pulse INTERVAL and PULSE DURATION controls each are set at 1 msec and the identical procedure followed. A present or absent response to faradic current then is recorded.

Rheobase (Polar) Ratio and Rheobase

In the early days of EDX, emphasis was placed upon the use of the anode versus the cathode as the stimulating electrode to produce a contraction. With a constant amount of current, stimulation by the cathode produces a stronger contraction when the switch is closed (make) than when it is opened (break). Also, the closing contraction is greater when the cathode, instead of the anode, is employed (CCC > ACC > AOC > COC).* This rule does not find clinical application today except to emphasize that the cathode should be the electrode used for stimulation because anodal current may be of an intensity sufficient to cause pain and alter the response. Uniformity of reporting results is necessary, and the routine use of the cathode as the stimulating electrode permits this.

The polar or rheobase ratio refers to the anode closing contraction in milliamperes, divided by the corresponding value for the cathode closing contraction in milliamperes. In denervation, muscle becomes more sensitive to these currents, causing a reversal of polarity; thus, the anode is equally effective as the cathode in causing contraction. A normal polar ratio is over 1.5, and this drops to 1.0 or less in denervation.

The rheobase (anode and/or cathode) is determined in a manner analogous to location of the motor point (q.v.). By definition, the rheobase, or utilization time, is the least amount of current which, flowing for an "infinite" period of time, is just sufficient to cause minimal contraction of muscle. The rheobase is rather variable from muscle to muscle in the same and opposite limbs (4 to 8 ma) so that, taken by itself, it is not a useful diagnostic tool. However, it forms the basis for the determination of the polar ratio, chronaxie, and strength-duration curve, and therefore must be determined accurately for the muscle in question. Once the motor point has been located, the PULSE DURATION control is set at 300 msec (which is considered "infinite time" for muscle), and single pulses are delivered to the muscle. The INTENSITY control then is turned clockwise so that the current is increased slowly from zero to that value which causes minimum twitch of muscle. By switching polarity from cathode to anode, the value for the anode and cathode rheobase can be determined (Fig. 4–3). The polar, or rheobase, ratio is then calculated. This parameter need not be included in routine clinical EDX.

Strength-Duration (S-D) Curve

If the interval between pulses and the current at rheobase level both are held constant, the duration of each pulse can be shortened progressively until the

*Cathodal closing contraction is greater than anodal closing contraction is greater than anodal opening contraction is greater than cathodal opening contraction.

current is too brief to cause contraction. This will vary from muscle to muscle, but at some point (for example, 3 msec) the current duration will be too brief to cause response. To do so, current strength must be increased. If pulse duration is shortened still further, it eventually will be too brief to cause any contraction, no matter how strong the current is. An S-D curve consists of plotting the pulse duration (milliseconds) against current (milliamperes) necessary to cause minimum contraction at each of several pulse durations, holding the pulse interval constant (Figs. 4–3 and 4–4). Referring to a standard logarithmic chart of an S-D curve (Fig. 5–4), the rheobase lies at the lower right corner. Once this has been determined, it is plotted on the chart. Leaving the electrode on the motor point and the current the same (for example, 5 ma, the rheobase), the PULSE DURATION control is turned to a shorter pulse duration, 100 msec. At this new pulse duration, it can be noted at once whether contractions are present. Because pulse interval is immaterial and the observation time at each control setting may be a matter of several seconds, it may be more comfortable for the patient to deliver single pulses from the machine, rather than a pulse every second. This is accomplished by setting the SELECTOR switch at SINGLE IMPULSE. These single pulses can be delivered either from the machine itself or from the foot pedal on the floor, as noted earlier.

If contractions are seen at the new, shorter duration setting, the PULSE DURATION control is turned to 50, 30, 10, 5, 4, and 3 msec, in that order, with the required milliamperes of current plotted at each setting. This is done until contractions no longer are present at a given pulse duration. At this point, the current is increased very slightly (in 0.5-ma increments) until contractions again appear. This point (current value in milliamperes) also is plotted on the chart, and the next briefer pulse duration is used. If contractions are not present, the current is increased again until they reappear, and this current value is plotted. This process is repeated until further current increase fails to produce contraction (impulses too brief). In a normal nerve-muscle preparation, this will occur as the left side of the S-D graph is approached, usually near 0.05 or 0.1 msec. The more points that are

Fig. 4–4. Strength duration curves. Evaluation: *1*, normal; *2*, partial denervation (discontinuous); *3*, complete denervation; *C*, chronaxie; *R*, rheobase (i.e., C_1, chronaxie for Curve 1; R_1, rheobase for Curve 1). Values are: R_1, 6 ma; R_2, 4 ma; R_3, 2 ma; C_1, 0.2 msec; C_2, 5.0 msec; C_3, 22 msec.

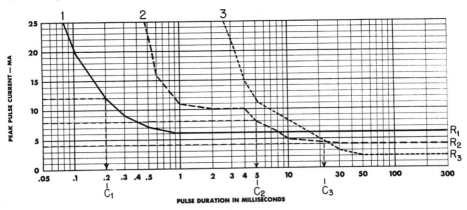

plotted on an S-D curve, the smoother and more accurate it will be. A compromise is obtained by plotting the following points: 300, 100, 50, 30, 10, 5, 4, 3, 2, 1, 0.5, 0.4, 0.3, 0.2, 0.1 and 0.05 msec. Fewer points can be used, depending upon the apparatus available. At each of these pulse durations, the amount of current required for minimum muscular contraction is noted and plotted on the graph. This produces a parabolic curve which is asymptotic.

Because a normal neuromuscular preparation is sensitive to currents of very brief duration, the curve will begin to rise toward the left side of the graph. Increased current will be required only when the duration of impulses becomes very short (Fig. 4–4). On the other hand, if the muscle is denervated, it behaves as "muscle alone" and therefore is insensitive to currents of brief duration; the curve rises sharply toward the right side of the graph. If there is partial denervation, or reinnervation, the S-D curve will rise somewhere between the two extremes and may have one or more discontinuities or "bumps," which correspond to the algebraic sum of the nerve and muscle curves just described (Fig. 4–4). The S-D curve is most useful in following regeneration or progressive denervation of a muscle, because serial studies will demonstrate shifts of the curve toward or away from normality.

Chronaxie

Used as a means of estimating the slope of the S-D curve rapidly, chronaxie is defined arbitrarily as the time required for an amount of current twice rheobasic strength to cause minimum contraction of muscle. On a normal S-D curve (Fig. 4–4), the point at which a current twice rheobasic strength intersects the curve will fall well under 1 msec. Any chronaxie value over 1.0 msec is abnormal, indicating a shift of the curve toward the right. This value rises in denervation and falls toward normal in reinnervation. The chronaxie may be determined after the S-D curve has been plotted simply by doubling the rheobase and finding the point (in milliseconds) at which this milliampere value intersects the S-D curve (Fig. 4–4). However, the chronaxie may be determined separately (before the S-D curve is plotted) as soon as the rheobase has been determined. This is done by leaving the stimulating electrode in place over the motor point and doubling the rheobase by turning the SELECTOR switch to CHRON. (Fig. 4–3). The PULSE DURATION vernier control is turned to 0.05 msec, the duration is increased by successive steps until minimum muscle twitch is observed, and this value is then recorded as the chronaxie and should be under 1 msec. However, the chronaxie alone is not as useful as the entire S-D curve, because one or more discontinuities may be observed in instances in which the chronaxie is normal.

Repetitive-Stimulus (R-S) or Strength-Interval (S-I) Curve

The S-I curve is synonymous with the R-S curve. It may be used as an adjunctive procedure, though it need not form an integral part of routine clinical EDX. When stimuli of constant duration are quite close together in time, they tend to summate, to produce contraction, even though each individual impulse would not be effective. This phenomenon is more marked in a normal muscle than in one which is denervated, because normal muscle responds more readily to stimuli of short duration. The S-I curve may be plotted on a graph identical to the S-D curve, except that the values on the abscissa will refer to pulse interval rather than pulse

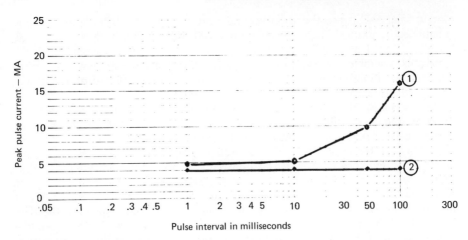

Fig. 4–5. Strength interval curves. **1.** Abnormal (ascending) S–I curve, rising in the right portion where no summation of brief stimuli is possible. **2.** Normal (flat) S–I curve. S–I curves may be plotted on same form as S–D curves (Fig. 4–4); however, abscissa represents pulse duration in S–D and pulse interval in S–I curves.

duration. In contrast to an S-D curve, where pulse interval is immaterial and pulse duration is varied and recorded, the S-I curve employs a variable interval while the duration is held constant. The pulses used are 1.0 msec in duration, beginning the curve with a pulse interval of 1.0 msec. The current is increased gradually until minimum muscle contraction is observed. This value is plotted on the S-I curve (Fig. 4-5). The interval between pulses is then progressively lengthened. For convenience, four additional points of curve are selected: 10–, 50–, and 100–msec intervals. Milliamperes of current values are plotted for each point. In normal muscle, no increase in current is required, even though the interval between stimuli is progressively lengthened. This results in a straight-line curve. However, in denervation, more current will be required as the interval lengthens, because muscle alone is insensitive to currents of such brief duration, and no summation is possible when long pulse intervals are used. Thus, the curve will rise to the right side, a so-called "ascending" S-I curve (Fig. 4-5).

Galvanic Tetanus Ratio (GTR)

Tetanus is defined as contraction of muscle which persists after cessation of the stimulus. It can be demonstrated when testing for response to galvanic current. When the switch is closed, a brief twitch of muscle will occur but, as the current is raised, a point will be reached when the contraction persists. This will occur both on the make and break of the circuit. The determination of the exact milliampere value for tetanus as opposed to isolated muscle twitch is often difficult and may be somewhat painful. However, after obtaining the rheobase, which may be defined for this purpose as the intensity of current required to reach "galvanic threshold," the current is increased progressively until there is no longer a simple muscle twitch but rather a sustained contraction after cessation of the stimulus. Normally, approximately three times the amount of current required for rheobase is needed to produce tetanus. Denervated muscle is much more irritable and therefore exhibits tetanus at currents which are the same as, or perhaps only slightly greater than, rheobase strength. If one divides the amount of current required for tetanus by the amount required for rheobase, the GTR is obtained. This is normally 3.0 or higher and falls to 1.0 in denervation. In reinnervation, the GTR rises again to its normal value of 3.0 or more.

ARTIFACTS AND SOURCES OF ERROR

Dry Electrodes

Because the EDX procedure may last several minutes or more, the electrodes may dry out in the air, resulting in poor conductivity. This condition will produce erroneous values, because higher currents will be needed to produce a minimum twitch. No response at all may be obtained even when very high currents are used, and the patient will complain of pain. The electrodes should be inspected often to insure that they are well moistened at all times.

Loose Connections

The milliammeter dial may register current being delivered when no visible responses are obtained, even with high currents. In this event, all wires should be checked for proper connection and all switches for the correct settings.

Pathological Conditions in Which Testing Is Difficult

Edema of subcutaneous tissue may produce high skin resistance, causing the current value not to reflect the actual amount required for muscle contraction. In denervation, the motor point may enlarge so that a careful examination is necessary before the correct value for rheobase is accepted.

Incorrect Lighting

Experience will dictate the end point for minimum muscle twitch. This will vary with the lighting used. The latter should be adequate and constant throughout the examination.

Moving the Electrodes

The stimulating electrode should be held in a constant position during the test. If it is moved away from the motor point, the S-D curve will alter as the threshold changes.

Voluntary Contraction of Muscle

In certain tense individuals, voluntary contraction of the muscle being tested may be confused with the evoked response. In these instances, the test is difficult to interpret. Fasciculations in disease states may produce similar difficulties. Observation of the flashing of the indicator lamp on the EDX unit will help to avoid this difficulty.

INTERPRETATION OF FINDINGS

Referring to Table 4–1, it can be seen that a normal pattern of response includes a positive response to both faradic and galvanic current, a rheobase ratio of more than 1.5, a rheobase of 5–8 ma (variable), a chronaxie less than 1.0 msec, an S-D curve which rises toward the left of the graph, a straight S-I curve, and a GTR of over 3.0. In total denervation, there is still a positive response to galvanic current, unless there has been complete atrophy of muscle, but faradic current produces no contraction. The rheobase ratio falls to less than 1.0, the rheobase usually falls (initially the muscle is more irritable), but may rise later as atrophy ensues. The chronaxie rises to over 1.0 msec., the S-D curve shifts to the right with discontinuities, the S-I curve ascends to the right, and the GTR approaches 1.0. These parameters find greatest application in cases of traumatic nerve injury when it is necessary to determine 1) the degree of denervation and 2) the course of recovery. Changes in these parameters usually appear within 1–3 weeks after clinical injury to a nerve, so testing prior to this time may fail to detect denervation. However, return toward normal may occur before clinical recovery takes place. The patient should be tested no more often than every week and no less frequently than every month until sufficient serial determinations have been made to establish the course of the lesion. Changes in the parameters toward normal are favorable, and the converse offers a bad prognosis. These studies also are used to differentiate upper from lower motor neuron diseases, but find little application in the study of muscular dystrophy, myotonia, and myasthenia gravis, where EMG is much more useful. In these diseases (diseases of muscle and the neuromuscular junction), EDX studies are normal, excluding those cases in which severe atrophy or fatigability of muscle prohibits an adequate test.

The S-D curve, as well as the other parameters discussed, are normal in cases of hysterical paralysis and in upper motor neuron lesions.

SUMMARY OF STEPS IN ROUTINE CLINICAL ELECTRODIAGNOSIS

Step 1. Turn on the machine and allow it to warm up. During this time, familiarize yourself with the patient's history and physical findings. Introduce yourself to the patient and proceed with any necessary history and/or neurologic examination.

Step 2. Explain the test to the patient as described in Chapter 2.

Step 3. Position the patient appropriately so that the limb to be tested is at complete rest and is well illuminated by either room or oblique lighting from a floor lamp.

Step 4. Electrodiagnostic studies are accomplished best when one person assists the examiner by recording the findings as the test proceeds. A printed chart is available with most units (Fig. 4–4).

Step 5. Moisten the indifferent electrode (gauze wire mesh) with saline or water so that it is soaked thoroughly. Dry the outside gently with a gauze sponge. Connect the indifferent electrode to the appropriate lead wire and the stimulating electrode to the other outlet. Soak the felt of the stimulating electrode with saline. Connect the indifferent electrode and stimulating electrode wires to the machine, and position the polarity switch so that the stimulating electrode is the cathode (Figs. 4–2 and 4–3).

Step 6. After the patient has been positioned, seat yourself comfortably next to the patient so that **both** of you are relaxed. Proceed to locate the motor point of the muscle. Place the indifferent electrode on the same extremity as the muscle being tested, and the stimulating electrode over the approximate location of the motor point as determined from a suitable chart.[1]

Step 7. Set the OUTPUT switch on SINGLE IMPULSE, the current dial at 0.5 milliampere, and the SELECTOR switch at RHEO. 300 msec (pulse duration).

Step 8. Proceed as instructed above for the determination of rheobase, chronaxie, and S-D curve, recording the results on the appropriate chart.

Step 9. If the response of the muscle seems atypical, test a control muscle in a homologous area on the opposite side for comparison.

Step 10. Proceed with any other muscles to be studied.

REFERENCES

1.Light S: Electrodiagnosis and Electromyography, 2nd ed. Baltimore, Waverly Press, 1961

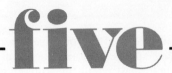

REPORTING RESULTS WITH ILLUSTRATIVE CASE REPORTS

The electroneuromyographer has several functions, only one of which is the actual performance of the test. He must 1) perform an adequate, accurate, and efficient study and then 2) identify the disturbance in degree and location. Based on these data, he then will 3) provide clinical correlation using both ENM and clinical data, and 4) report these findings and interpretations in a clear and understandable fashion. This formulation takes place before the patient leaves the laboratory.

The electroneuromyographer will find that each facet of ENM—NSS, EMG, and EDX—has both special and general application, depending on the nature of the clinical problem. He must decide which units are appropriate to the specific situation. For example, in a patient with myasthenia gravis, repetitive stimulation (to detect a junctional defect) and EMG will be most appropriate. A traumatic lesion of a peripheral nerve will require NCV measurements to locate the site of the lesion and its extent, and EDX to follow the progress of recovery. If anterior horn cell involvement is suspected (e.g., amyotrophic lateral sclerosis), NSS and EMG will be required. In complex problems such as a patient with diabetes mellitus, all three techniques may be required. Table 5–1 presents characteristic patterns of alterations of ENM parameters which result from involvement at various anatomic locations along the nerve muscle pathways.

The experienced electroneuromyographer approaches the examination in problem-solving fashion, not only at the conclusion of the examination but during the entire procedure. The extent and nature of what he does is designed to verify or exclude tentative hypotheses that are formed on an ongoing basis. For example, in a patient with a suspect carpal tunnel syndrome, the finding of a prolonged distal latency of the median nerve is not sufficient. The experienced electroneuromyographer will search for abnormal findings *above* the wrist to be sure that a root/plexus lesion is not presenting as a carpal tunnel syndrome.

In a case of suspected cervical spondylosis, the finding of denervation potentials in the arms is only a partial answer. Experience dictates that muscles in the lower extremities should be examined, because amyotrophic lateral sclerosis is part of the differential diagnosis. Thus, ENM becomes an extension of the neurologic examination and never should be a diagnostic procedure divorced from problem-solving techniques. The physician performing the study as well as the clinician must be aware that negative findings on the ENM do not exclude the presence of disease.

An appropriate requisition completed by the referring source should accompany each patient. In this way, the electroneuromyographer can become familiar with the problem with which he is confronted. However, this requisition is only a prelude, and additional information in the form of history and neurologic examination always is required. For purposes of brevity, the requisitions pertinent to the cases in this chapter have been omitted. ENM worksheets are presented in each case to follow, but are abridged to conserve space. Upon completion of the study, the findings and conclusions are reported on an appropriate form. A copy of each report is kept on file in the laboratory and another is sent to the referring source. Careful documentation and record keeping is important for both teaching and medicolegal purposes.

In the total evaluation of a given patient, the sequence of the studies is important. For example, in a patient who complains of weakness, the initial step is a careful history and physical examination. This will provide, among other items, information regarding the distribution and nature of the weakness. In general, the order of subsequent studies is as follows:

1. Blood and urine chemistry studies
2. Cerebrospinal fluid examination (may be performed at the time of myelography)
3. ENM
4. Myelography, if indicated
5. Muscle (nerve) biopsy (avoid sites studied by EMG)

A series of case presentations in this chapter illustrate the application of ENM techniques to the study of diseases which affect various segments along the peripheral neuromuscular pathway. In each case, the history and clinical findings will be followed by pertinent laboratory data. Representative ENM records from that case are illustrated, together with the final report. Finally, interpretation of the ENM findings is discussed in the context of the overall picture. The final section is devoted to ENM problem-solving. Five ENM exercises are presented, which allow the reader to form his own interpretation from the available data before clinical history, neurologic findings, and the authors' clinical correlation are given. Some of the cases presented appeared in the first edition of this manual. Each has been reviewed and additional data have been made available wherever possible.

In some instances, data are missing which, in retrospect, would have been helpful in the ENM formulation. As is often the case in actual practice, such data are wanted in retrospect and the patient must be retested at a later date. We will point out such omissions as they occur from case to case. Abbreviations which have not been explained elsewhere include: N = normal (e.g., for percentage of polyphasic MUP, N = less than 10%). 0 = none observed. I and D refer to increased and decreased, respectively. M = myotonic discharge.

Table 5-1. ENM—LOCATION OF LESION WITH REPRESENTATIVE DISORDERS

Parameter	Functional Syndromes Hysteria	Upper Motor Neuron Lesion Cerebro-vascular Accident	Neurono-pathies Poliomyelitis, Amotrophic Lateral Sclerosis	Neurono-pathy–Neuropathy Peroneal Muscular Atrophy
A. Nerve Stimulation Studies				
1. Motor: NCV	Normal	Normal	Normal or slightly decreased	Decreased
2. Motor: Latency	Normal	Normal	Normal	Prolonged
3. Sensory: Latency	Normal	Normal	Normal	Prolonged
B. Electromyography				
1. Insertion Potentials	Normal	Normal	Increased	Increased
2. Resting Potentials				
a. Fibrillation and Positive waves	None	None	Present	Present
b. Fasciculations	None	None	Present–marked	Present
3. Voluntary Contraction–MUP				
a. Amplitude MUP	Normal	Normal	Increased	Increased
b. Duration MUP	Normal	Normal	Increased	Increased
c. Number/Strength[1]	Normal	Normal	Normal or slightly reduced	Normal or slightly reduced
d. Total number	Normal	Reduced	Reduced	Reduced
e. Polyphasic MUP, number and (size)	Normal	Slightly increased	Increased (large)	Increased
f. Rate of firing	Irregular	Usually decreased	Usually decreased	Normal or decreased
C. Electrodiagnosis: S–D Curve	Normal	Normal	Denervation	Denervation
D. Remarks	Bizarre voluntary patterns		Rare type II myotonic discharges	Findings vary with anatomic sites involved

1. Number of MUP relative to strength of contraction.
2. May be decreased with multiple root involvement.

	Neuropathies			Neuromyal Junction	Myopthies	
	Herniated Nucleus Pulposus	Diabetic Neuropathy	Carpal Tunnel Syndrome	Myasthenia Gravis	Polymyositis	Duchenne Muscular Dystrophy
Normal[2]	Decreased	Normal or slightly decreased	Normal	Normal	Normal
Normal	Prolonged	Normal	Normal	Normal	Normal
Normal	Prolonged	Prolonged	Normal	Normal	Normal
Increased	Increased slightly	Increased	Normal	Increased	Normal
Present	Present	Present	None	Present	None or rare
Rare	None or rare	None or rare	None	None	None
Normal	Normal	Normal	Varying	Reduced	Reduced
Normal	Normal	Normal	Normal	Reduced	Reduced
Normal	Normal	Normal	Normal	Increased	Increased
Reduced slightly	Reduced	Reduced	Reduced with fatigue	Decreased late	Decreased late
Increased	Increased	Increased	Normal	Increased (small)	Increased (small)
Normal	Normal	Normal	Tends to decline	Rapid	Rapid
Denervation	Denervation	Denervation	Normal	Relatively normal	Normal
Type II myotonic potentials can be seen	Sensory conduction slow before motor	Increased latency through compression zone is hallmark	Repetitive stimulation shows decrement of evoked response	Type I or II myotonic discharges	Type I myotonic discharges in myoonic dystrophy

FUNCTIONAL

Case 1

COMPENSATION NEUROSIS (Hysteria)

I. HISTORY.   While working at his job on a railroad, a 45-year-old male pulled a switch. The lever seemed to "slip out of his hand"; the next thing he knew, the switch was "released." That night his back and neck felt sore, and he experienced discomfort in his shoulders. The pain developed and increased rapidly so that he hardly could move. Despite various and persistent treatment, the pain remained constant over the next two years.

II. PHYSICAL FINDINGS
   A. *General physical examination.* Normal.
   B. *Neurologic examination.*
      1. *Mental status and language.* The patient appeared quite apprehensive and the examiner questioned whether full cooperation was being given.
      2. *Cranial nerves.* No deficits.
      3. *Motor.* When individual muscles were tested, the patient rarely exerted full strength and would suddenly "let go." Voluntary neck movement was slow and labored but, given time, neck movements seemed free in all directions without pain. On palpation, however, the nuchal muscles were tight and tender.
      4. *Reflexes.* The muscle-stretch reflexes were brisk and equal. There was no Hoffmann sign. The abdominal reflexes were brisk and equal and there were no pathological reflexes.
      5. *Coordination.* No deficits.
      6. *Sensation.* There was no sensory loss to any modality, including pain, touch, vibration, and joint sense.

III. LABORATORY DATA.   X rays of the skull, cervical vertebrae, and chest were normal. A cervical myelogram was performed. On the cross-table lateral film, evidence of minimal-posterior bar formation was noted at the lower cervical interspaces. This was interpreted as normal for his age. The examination of the cerebrospinal fluid likewise was normal.

IV. CLINICAL IMPRESSION.   Compensation neurosis (Hysteria).

V. ENM
   A. *NERVE STIMULATION STUDIES (NSS).*

Nerve		LATENCY (msec)				NCV (m/sec)	
		Motor		Sensory			
			N		N		N
L	Ulnar	3.4	2.3-3.4			58.0	49-66
R	Ulnar	3.3	2.3-3.4			59.0	49-66
L	Median	4.4	2.7-4.2			58.0	48-68
R	Median	4.2	2.7-4.2			57.5	48.68

B. *ELECTROMYOGRAPHY (EMG).*

L or R	MUSCLE	INSERTION ACTIVITY	POTENTIALS AT REST			MOTOR UNIT POTENTIALS (MUP)				
						Individual MUP			Interference	
			Fib	Pos Waves	Fas	dur (msec)	amp (mV)	% poly-phasic	Pat	amp (mV)
L	Abductor digiti II	N	0	0	0	6-8	1.5	N	3+	2.5
R	Deltoid	N	0	0	0	3-5	1.5	N	3+	2.0
R	Biceps brachii	N	0	0	0	4-6	2.0	N	3+	2.5
R	Supraspinatus	N	0	0	0	5-8	1.5	N	3+	2.0

C. *SUMMARY OF FINDINGS AND CLINICAL SIGNIFICANCE. NSS.* Normal. *EMG.* Normal parameters of individual MUPs. The recruitment pattern during voluntary contraction was bizarre and inconstant. The number of MUPs, however, was consistent with the strength of contraction. The patient did not make a maximal effort, so that the examiner could not assess full interference pattern.

Normal ENM study, which did not reveal any defect of the motor unit. The bizarre and inconstant recruitment pattern is compatible with the clinical impression of a functional syndrome.

VI. COMMENT. The absence of fibrillation potentials or other significant abnormality in the muscles tested argues against an organic lesion in the lower motor neuron. The ENM correlate of the clinical pattern of inconstant voluntary muscle contraction was intermittent bursts of MUPs, each one of which, however, was within normal limits with regard to duration, amplitude and waveform. Nerve conduction velocities likewise were normal, a finding against a multiple-root lesion in the neck or peripheral nerve damage.

Electroneuromyography can perform a valuable service both from the medical and legal standpoints in cases of suspected malingering, hysteria, and compensation neurosis when combined with a careful examination. Cases exist in which pronounced functional overlay masks an underlying organic substrate. ENM offers an objective approach to the problem, an attempt to establish the presence of organic pathology. The converse is also true, and ENM forms an important medicolegal tool in such cases.

UPPER MOTOR NEURON LESION

Case 2

CEREBROVASCULAR ACCIDENT

I. HISTORY. A 58-year-old grocery salesman was brought to the emergency room of a hospital by his wife, who said that he awoke that morning unable to speak or move the right arm or leg. The patient had suffered from hypertension for about 12 years and had taken medication sporadically. His blood pressure 3 months prior to admission was 180/110. For several months, he had complained of brief periods of numbness in the right arm and leg, accompanied by some difficulty in speaking. He had not notified his doctors of this problem, because he attributed it to "nerves." His past history was unremarkable. The family history indicated that his father had died of a "stroke."

II. PHYSICAL FINDINGS

A. *General physical examination.* On examination in the emergency room, his blood pressure was 164/100, pulse 88, and respirations 22. There was a minimal systolic murmur at the apex of the heart, and a faint bruit was detected over the left carotid artery.

B. Neurologic examination

1. *Mentalstatusandlanguage.* There was a profound expressive aphasia. Although the patient was able to follow commands, he was unable to utter a word.
2. *Cranial nerves.* Right central VII nerve weakness.
3. *Motor.* Flaccid right hemiplegia.
4. *Reflexes.* The muscle-stretch reflexes on the right were lost uniformly. There was no Hoffmann sign, but there was a strong right Babinski sign.
5. *Coordination.* No deficits other than where limited by paralysis.
6. *Sensation.* No demonstrable deficits.

A left carotid arteriogram revealed complete occlusion of the left internal carotid artery in the neck and a carotid endarterectomy was performed.

Over the next several weeks, the patient's blood pressure was controlled with antihypertensive medication. He was given physiotherapy, speech therapy, and occupational therapy. There was some return of speech over the next several months. He was able to walk with a minimum of assistance, but very little function returned to the right arm. Six months after the initial deficit, he seemed to understand most of what was spoken but continued to have some difficulty speaking and had little use of the right hand.

III. LABORATORY DATA.

The following studies were found to be normal at the time of admission: CBC, sedimentation rate, BUN, creatinine, FBS, electrolytes, alkaline and acid phosphatase, SGOT, LDH, SGPT, serology, urinalysis, and ECG. Uric acid was at the upper limits of normal, and chest X ray revealed slight cardiomegaly. An intravenous pyelogram was normal. Cerebrospinal fluid examination on the day following admission revealed 4 WBC; 3 RBC; protein, 50 mg%; sugar, 85 mg%; chloride, 94 mEq/liter; negative serology; and normal electrophoresis.

IV. CLINICAL IMPRESSION.

Occlusion of the left internal carotid artery with infarction in the distribution of the left middle cerebral artery with right hemiplegia and aphasia.

V. ENM

A. *NERVE STIMULATION STUDIES (NSS).*

Skin temperature = 33°C

Nerve		LATENCY (msec)				NCV (m/sec)	
		Motor		Sensory			
		N		N			N
R	Median	4.1	2.7-4.2	3.6	2.3-3.2	47.0	48-68
R	Ulnar	3.6	2.3-3.4	3.4	2.1-3.0	46.0	49-66

B. *ELECTROMYOGRAPHY (EMG).*

L or R	MUSCLE	INSERTION ACTIVITY	POTENTIALS AT REST			MOTOR UNIT POTENTIALS (MUP)				
						Individual MUP			Interference	
			Fib	Pos Waves	Fas	dur (msec)	amp (mV)	% poly-phasic	Pat	amp (mV)
R	Abductor digiti quinti	N	0	0	0	5-10	1-2	N	3+	2
R	Abductor pollicis brevis	N	0	1+	0	5-10	1-2	N	3+	2
R	First Dorsal Interosseus	N	1+	1+	0	5-10	1-2	N	3+	2
R	Flexar pollicis brevis	N	1+	1+	0	"	"	N	3+	2
R	Biceps	N	0	0	0	"	"	N	3+	2
R	Deltoid	N	0	0	0	"	"	N	3+	2
L	First Dorsal Interosseus	N	0	0	0	"	"	N	3+	2
L	Abductor pollicis brevis	N	0	0	0	"	"	N	3+	2
L	Triceps	N	0	0	0	"	"	N	3+	2

C. *SUMMARY OF FINDINGS AND CLINICAL SIGNIFICANCE. NSS.*
Borderline NCV study of the right median nerve and slightly slow NCV of the right ulnar nerve. Sensory latencies prolonged in both nerves tested; motor latency of right ulnar nerve prolonged. *EMG.* Fibrillations observed in the right first dorsal interosseous and flexor pollicis brevis muscles, and a few positive waves seen in the right abductor pollicis brevis. Individual MUPs were normal. Interference pattern normal.

The slightly slow NCV values may be related to the reduced temperature of the extremity (33° C) compared with the opposite side (35° C). The EMG pattern was of no definite diagnostic pattern. A repeat EMG is recommended at the clinician's discretion in 2–4 months.

VI. COMMENT.
This patient's history and physical finding at the time of admission to the hospital together with the subsequent course all indicate a cerebrovascular accident. Because of the return of speech and use of the lower

extremity and shoulder, further information was sought for the reason for lack of return of adequate hand function. The ENM findings of slightly decreased nerve conduction velocities of the median and ulnar nerves are interpreted as due to decreased temperature of the extremity (affected side: 33° C, normal side 35° C). The scattered denervation potentials could not be correlated with a lower motor neuron lesion and were considered nondiagnostic. The recommendation that the study be repeated 2–4 months was not carried out.

Such minimal findings on the ENM study must be interpreted with caution. Unless the examiner can make a definitive statement based on well-documented findings, broad interpretations should not be made.

NEURONOPATHY

Case 3

AMYOTROPHIC LATERAL SCLEROSIS

I. HISTORY. A 51-year-old white male machinist was admitted to the hospital with a history of difficulty walking for 3 years. The problem began insidiously with pain in both knees, low-back tenderness over the coccyx, and an unsteady gait. Ever since, walking has been a problem; he found it increasingly difficult to walk on his tiptoes and heels. X rays of the lumbar spine were reported as normal 3 years ago.

For 10 years, he had complained of pain and stiffness in the shoulders; x-ray studies revealed calcification in the supraspinatus tendon on the right.

One year prior to admission, a myelogram showed partial obstruction at the T11–12 level, with a definite defect on the right side. A laminectomy had been performed. The findings at operation were reported as "circumscribed arachnoiditis."

II. PHYSICAL FINDINGS
  A. *General physical examination.* No abnormalities.
  B. *Neurological examination*
    1. *Mental status and language.* Intact.
    2. *Cranial nerves.* There was moderate dysarthria (slurring of words). The left side of the face was weak, but the forehead wrinkled equally well on the two sides. The extraocular movements were normal. There was no nystagmus. There was no weakness or atrophy of the tongue. The uvula moved in the midline and jaw strength was normal.
    3. *Motor.* Fasciculations were present bilaterally in the interosseus and plantar muscles. There was significant bilateral atrophy of the shoulder girdle muscles (Fig. 5–1). The lower extremities were spastic, with patellar clonus bilaterally. There was no ankle clonus. Muscle strength in the upper extremities was good except for weakness of the interosseus muscles, and there was slight falling away (drift) of the right upper extremity. He could walk on toe and heel on both sides to some extent but could not hop on either foot.

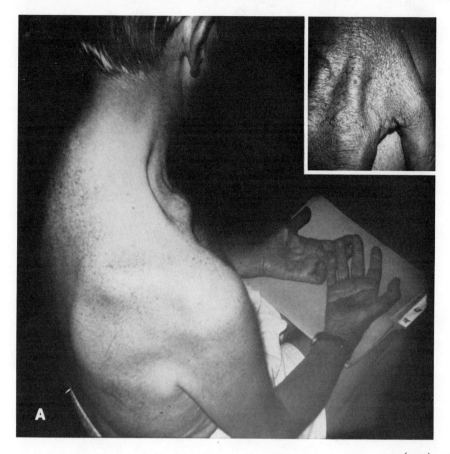

(continued)

Fig. 5–1. Case 3. Neuronopathy. Amyotrophic lateral sclerosis. **A.** Photograph of patient with amyotrophic lateral sclerosis, showing focal atrophy of the supra- and infraspinatus muscles and the small muscles of the hands. **B.** Muscle biopsy showing neurogenic (grouped) atrophy. Grouped atrophic fibers within muscle bundles with many angulated fibers present. Courtesy Dr. E. R. Ross. (H & E, ×125).

4. *Reflexes.* The muscle-stretch reflexes were symmetrical throughout, except that the right knee jerk was greater than the left. There was a left Hoffmann sign, none on the right. The plantar responses were flexor when the sole of the foot was stimulated, but there were bilateral Gonda responses. The abdominal reflexes were brisk and equal.
5. *Coordination.* No deficits.
6. *Sensation.* Intact.

III. LABORATORY DATA.   Hematocrit, 40%; WBC, 10,300; FBS, 75 mg%; EEG, nonspecific, mild generalized abnormal. X ray of the chest was normal; thoracic spine films revealed scoliosis convex to the right, with slight wedging

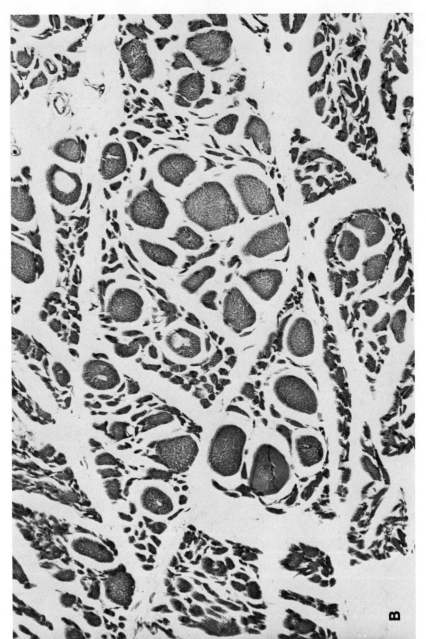

Fig. 5-1 B.

and marginal irregularities involving the mid-thoracic bodies. The disc spaces were intact, with a suggestion of slight residual deformity secondary to juvenile epiphysitis of the lower thoracic vertebral bodies. The myelogram was repeated. It showed an obstruction of the flow of contrast material at the level of T10—T11, and a defect in the laminae of T11 and T12. The nature of this defect could not be determined. The cerebrospinal fluid findings at the time of myelography were within normal limits: cell count, 1 lymphocyte; protein, 30 mg%; serology, negative; electrophoresis, normal.

IV. CLINICAL IMPRESSION.   Amyotrophic lateral sclerosis.

V. ENM
A. NERVE STIMULATION STUDIES (NSS).

		LATENCY (msec)				NCV (m/sec)	
		Motor		Sensory			
	Nerve		N		N		N
L	Median	3.7	2.7-4.2			59.0	48-68
R	Median	3.3	2.7-4.2			57.3	48-68
L	Peroneal	3.9	3.7-6.1			46.8	44-58
R	Peroneal	3.9	3.7-6.1			46.2	44-58

B. ELECTROMYOGRAPHY (EMG).

L or R	MUSCLE	INSERTION ACTIVITY	POTENTIALS AT REST			MOTOR UNIT POTENTIALS (MUP)				
						Individual MUP			Interference	
			Fib	Pos Waves	Fas	dur (msec)	amp (mV)	% poly-phasic	Pat	amp (mV)
R	Deltoid	N	0	0	0	5-8	3	N	3+	6
L	Deltoid	N	0	0	0	"	3	N	2+	6
R	First Dorsal Interosseus	N	1+	1+	1+	"	5	N	2+	6
L	First Dorsal Interosseus	N	1+	1+	1+	"	5	N	2+	6
R	Quadriceps	N	1+	0	1+	"	2-3	N	2+	6
R	Tibialis anterior	N	0	0	1+	"	4	N	2+	6
L	Quadriceps	N	0	0	1+	"	3	N	2+	6
L	Tibialis anterior	N	1+	1+	1+	"	5	N	2+	6
L	Gastrocnemius	N	1+	1+	1+	"	5	N	1+	6
R	Tongue	N	1+	0	0	"	3	N	3+	6

C. SUMMARY OF FINDINGS AND CLINICAL SIGNIFICANCE.   NSS.
Normal. *EMG.* Numerous scattered fasciculations and fibrillations and positive waves in muscles of all four extremities (Fig. 5–2A, B and C) and tongue. MUPs were generally of normal duration, but increased amplitude (Fig. 5–2D). The interference pattern on maximal effort was reduced.

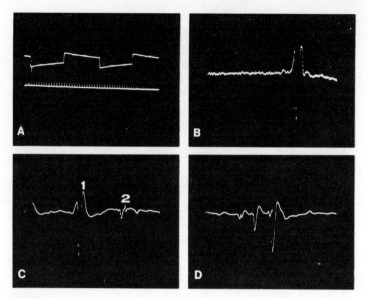

Fig. 5–2. Case 3. Neuronopathy. Amyotrophic lateral sclerosis. **A.** Calibration and time base for all recordings, co-axial needle electrodes: for B, 50 μV; for C, 100 μV; for D, 1 mV, 1 msec/div. **B.** Fasciculation recorded at rest from left gastrocnemius muscle. **C.** Fasciculation *(1)* and fibrillation *(2)* recorded at rest from left gastrocnemius muscle. **D.** Giant MUP on maximum effort recorded from right tibialis anterior.

       The ENM findings are compatible with diffuse anterior horn cell involvement.

VI. COMMENT. The normal NCV values and latencies in the face of fibrillation potentials in many muscles suggest that the pathology does not lie in the peripheral nerves or in the ventral roots, but rather in the anterior horn cell. The infrequent but giant voluntary action potentials and the fasciculations seen throughout also point to this conclusion. The significant ENM findings, the most revealing of which is the EMG, are compatible with a generalized process, most likely a diffuse neuronopathy. When viewed against this background, the mid-thoracic spinal cord lesion is not adequate to explain the neurologic symptoms and signs. The diagnosis of amyotrophic lateral sclerosis, probable from both clinical and ENM standpoints, best fits the progressive protracted course of the illness.

Case 4

SYRINGOMYELIA

I. HISTORY. For 4 months, this 15-year-old boy had noted "loss of feeling" in his left upper extremity. He described this as inability to perceive heat and cold; on several occasions, he had burned his left hand without realizing it. On closer questioning, he admitted that these symptoms may have been present earlier, but he had paid no attention to them. No family history of a similar illness was elicited; no history of trauma was given. The problem seemed to be slowly progressive, but the patient had experienced no great disability up to the time of examination.

II. PHYSICAL FINDINGS

A. *General physical examination.* There was marked kyphoscoliosis of the thoracic spine and exostoses of the left clavicle.

B. *Neurologic examination*

1. *Mental status and language.* No deficits.
2. *Cranial nerves.* Intact.
3. *Motor.* There was no definite weakness in the upper extremities, even to detailed muscle testing. Gait was likewise normal: He walked on toes and heels and climbed on a chair without difficulty. He hopped easily on either foot.
4. *Reflexes.* The muscle-stretch reflexes were brisk and symmetrical in the lower extremities, but equally diminished in the upper limbs. The left triceps and ulnar responses were absent, even with reinforcement. There was no Hoffmann sign. The plantar responses were flexor. The abdominal reflexes were absent bilaterally.
5. *Coordination.* No deficits.
6. *Sensation.* The sensory examination (Fig. 5–3A) revealed a suspended vest-like loss to pain and temperature over the entire left arm extending over the chest down to T9. On the right, pain and temperature loss extended from T3 to T10. Cotton touch, vibration, and joint sensations were intact. There was some questionable pain and temperature loss over the left side in the segment C3–C5 inclusive.

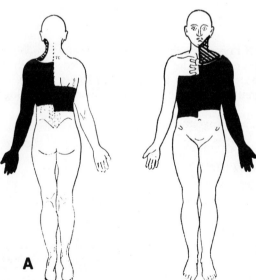

Fig. 5–3. Case 4. Neuronopathy. Syringomyelia. **A.** Sensory chart of case 4, showing suspended ("vest-like") sensory loss to pain and temperature (incomplete loss indicated by shaded area). **B.** Cervical myelogram, showing diffuse, fusiform enlargement of the cervical cord. Courtesy of Dr. E. Palacios.

A

(continued)

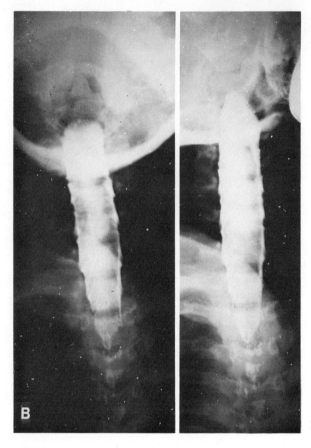

Fig. 5–3 B.

III. LABORATORY DATA.   X rays of the thoracic spine show kyphoscoliosis; films of the cervical spine were normal. The myelogram revealed symmetrical, fusiform enlargement of the cervical cord from C7 to T2 (Fig. 5–3B). The cerebrospinal fluid was normal (including cell count, protein, and serology).

IV. CLINICAL IMPRESSION.   Syringomyelia.

V. ENM
   A. *NERVE STIMULATION STUDIES (NSS)*.

	Nerve	LATENCY (msec)				NCV (m/sec)	
		Motor		Sensory			
			N		N		N
L	Ulnar	3.2	2.3-3.4	3.0	2.1-3.0	58.5	49-66
L	Median	3.7	2.7-4.2	3.2	2.3-3.2	55.0	48-68

B. *ELECTROMYOGRAPHY (EMG).*

L or R	MUSCLE	INSERTION ACTIVITY	POTENTIALS AT REST			MOTOR UNIT POTENTIALS (MUP)				
						Individual MUP			Interference	
			Fib	Pos Waves	Fas	dur (msec)	amp (mV)	% poly-phasic	Pat	amp (mV)
L	Deltoid	N	I+	I+	2+	5-10	5	N	3+	2
R	Deltoid	N	0	0	0	4-8	1	N	3+	2
L	Biceps brachii	N	I+	I+	0	6-10	.5	N	2+	1
R	Biceps brachii	N	0	0	0	4-6	1.5	N	3+	2
L	First Dorsal Interosseus	N	I+	0	I+	10-12	1-3	N	2+	.3
R	First Dorsal Interosseus	N	I+	0	0	4-6	1	N	3+	2
L	Paraspinal at T6	N	I+	I+	0	5-12	3	N	2+	3
L	Triceps	N	I+	I+	I+	5-12	3	N	2+	3
R	Triceps	N	I+	0	0	5-10	3	N	2+	3

C. *SUMMARY OF FINDINGS AND CLINICAL SIGNIFICANCE.   NSS.*
Within normal limits. *EMG:* Fibrillations and some fasciculations were
noted in muscles supplied by segments C5–T1 bilaterally. MUP relatively
normal.

These findings are compatible with a lower motor neuron lesion, C5–T1,
bilaterally, either at anterior horn cell and/or root level. An intramedullary
lesion of the spinal cord, C5–T1, could produce such a picture, but multiple
bilateral root involvement is also an adequate explanation.

VI. COMMENT.   Denervation potentials were seen in most muscles tested. Fasciculations also were noted. MUPs were relatively normal; no "giant" MUPs
typical of anterior horn cell involvement were observed, although some units
were as long as 12 msec and as high as 3 mV.

This pattern, together with normal NCV studies, suggests multiple root
and/or anterior horn cell involvement in the C5–T1 segments bilaterally. The
presence of fibrillations in the paraspinal muscles at T6 indicates 1) an extensive vertical lesion (C5–T6) and 2) a proximal lesion, i.e., anterior horn cell
and/or posterior root. Brachial plexus latency studies may help differentiate
an anterior horn cell from a root lesion, but the normal sensory latencies of
the median and ulnar nerves suggest that the lesion, at least for C7–C8, is
proximal to the sensory dorsal root ganglia.

Case 5.

ISCHEMIA OF THE SPINAL CORD **(Cervical spondylosis)**

I. HISTORY.   For the past 6 months, a 72-year-old female noted painless atrophy of the right hand without associated weakness. She denied sensory symptoms or any other disability. Specifically, cranial nerve functions were intact by
history, gait was unaffected, and the problem seemed relatively stable after she
first noticed it.

II. PHYSICAL FINDINGS

A. *General physical examination.* Unremarkable.

B. *Neurological examination*

1. *Mental status and language.* No deficits.
2. *Cranial nerves.* No deficits.
3. *Motor.* There was definite and profound atrophy of the right first dorsal interosseous muscle but very little of the right abductor digiti quinti. The same muscles were involved on the left, but the atrophy was less marked. The right thenar eminence was slightly atrophic, as were the deltoid muscles.
4. *Reflexes.* The muscle-stretch reflexes were diminished in the upper extremities. There was a left Babinski sign, none on the right.
5. *Coordination.* No deficits.
6. *Sensation.* No deficits.

III. LABORATORY DATA.
X ray of the chest was unremarkable. X ray of the cervical vertebrae revealed narrowing of the interspaces with spur formation impinging on the vertebral foramina at all levels. These changes were considered compatible with her age, and not sufficient to produce the symptoms described. A cervical myelogram was not performed, but examination of the cerebrospinal fluid was within normal limits, including cell count, protein, and serology.

IV. CLINICAL IMPRESSION.
Ischemia of the spinal cord as a consequence of cervical spondylosis.

V. ENM

A. *NERVE STIMULATION STUDIES (NSS).*

	Nerve	LATENCY (msec)				NCV (m/sec)	
		Motor		Sensory			
			N		N		N
L	Ulnar	2.8	2.3-3.4			62.0	49-66
R	Ulnar	2.8	2.3-3.4			49.4	49-66
L	Median	4.7	2.7-4.2			53.5	48-68
R	Median	3.7	2.7-4.2			51.5	48-68

B. ELECTROMYOGRAPHY (EMG).

L or R	MUSCLE	INSERTION ACTIVITY	POTENTIALS AT REST			MOTOR UNIT POTENTIALS (MUP)				
						Individual MUP			Interference	
			Fib	Pos Waves	Fas	dur (msec)	amp (mV)	% poly-phasic	Pat	amp (mV)
R	Deltoid	N	0	0	0	5-10	1.5	N	3+	2
R	Biceps brachii	I	1+	1+	1+	3-5	.5	Inc	3+	1
R	First Dorsal Interosseus	N	1+	0	1+	6-15	4.0	N	3+	4
L	First Dorsal Interosseus	N	1+	1+	1+	6-20	4.0	Inc	2+	4.5
R	Tibialis anterior	N	0	0	0	5	3.5	N	3+	2

C. SUMMARY OF FINDINGS AND CLINICAL SIGNIFICANCE.
NSS. Normal. Fibrillations, positive sharp waves and fasciculations noted
in the right biceps brachii and both first dorsal interosseus muscles. Some
of the MUPs were of prolonged duration and increased amplitude. Many
MUPs were polyphasic, some up to 20 msec duration.

The ENM findings are compatible with neuropathy with greatest involvement at the C8–T1 level.

VI. COMMENT.   The fibrillation potentials and the fasciculations seen in some
areas in both upper extremities confirm the presence of a lower motor neuron
lesion, but the normal nerve conduction velocity studies speak against multiple
root compression by cervical spondylosis as the cause of her problem. The
increased duration and amplitude of MUPs in some areas suggest the anterior
horn cell as the primary site of involvement. The presence of numerous polyphasic potentials, some of considerable duration, up to 20 msec, suggest an
ongoing denervative-reinnervative process.

The findings are in keeping with the clinical impression. Amyotrophic
lateral sclerosis was a consideration, but her age, the lack of progression, and
the lack of ENM involvement in the lower extremities even after many years
are against this diagnosis. The final clinical impression was ischemia of the
spinal cord with the brunt of involvement borne by the anterior horn cells in
the cervical area. This picture might result from compression of the anterior
spinal artery in cervical spondylosis.

Case 6.

WOHLFART-KUGELBERG-WELANDER (Chronic Proximal Spinal Muscular
Atrophy)

I. HISTORY.   A 57-year-old right-handed white male complained of weakness
in his arms and legs for 20 years. In 1941 he was rejected from military service
because he could not perform climbing, jumping, and running maneuvers. One
uncle had the same symptoms and two brothers are affected similarly. One
brother, N, 4 years younger, complained of loss of coordination and weakness
of his legs for 5 years prior to examination. On closer questioning, he was
uncertain as to whether the complaint may not have been present for many
years. The weakness had been slowly progressive. A second brother, J, in
adolesence at the time of examination (age 14), complained of some weakness
but the objective neurologic examination was unremarkable.

II. PHYSICAL FINDINGS
   A. *General physical examination.* No essential findings.
   B. *Neurologic examination*
      1. *Mental status and language.* Intact.
      2. *Cranial nerves.* Intact.
      3. *Motor.* On examination of the patient, there was marked foot drop
         bilaterally with a steppage gait. There was marked atrophy of the mus-
         cles of the lower extremities, especially below the knee. There was pro-
         nounced wasting of the interosseus muscles as well as atrophy of the
         more proximal muscles of the shoulder girdle. There were generalized

fasciculations (Fig. 5–4A). His brother, N, revealed a similar picture. There was a gait typical of bilateral foot drop. He was unable to walk on his toes or heels but could arise after squatting. There was both thenar and hypothenar atrophy.

4. *Reflexes.* Muscle-stretch reflexes were uniformly absent. There were no pathologic reflexes. His brother showed similar findings.
5. *Coordination.* No deficits.
6. *Sensation.* No deficits.

III. LABORATORY DATA.   Electroencephalography, brain scan, and skull X rays were within normal limits on all three brothers. X rays of the extremities of the two elder brothers showed a peculiar abnormality, diaphyseal aclasia. The ulna was forshortened, and there were osteochondromata involving the distal radius, ulna, and all the metacarpals. Both elbows revealed changes typical of multiple cartilagenous exostoses, with widening of the metaphyseal portion of the bone. The knees were similarly affected, and the ankles also revealed osteochondromata of the distal fibula and tibia. The joint spaces were well maintained. Serum enzymes on all three brothers were within normal limits, including LDH, SGOT, and CPK. Muscle biopsies were performed on the first two brothers, with findings typical of neurogenic atrophy.

IV. CLINICAL IMPRESSION.   Chronic proximal spinal muscular atrophy (Wohlfart–Kugelberg–Welander Disease).

V(a). ENM
   A. *NERVE STIMULATION STUDIES (NSS).*

Nerve		LATENCY (msec)			NCV (m/sec)	
		Motor		Sensory		
			N		N		N
R	Ulnar	3.5	2.3-3.4			52.9	49-66
R	Median	5.0	2.7-4.2			50.0	48-68
R	Peroneal	9.0	3.7-6.1			50.0	44-58

   B. *ELECTROMYOGRAPHY (EMG).*

L or R	MUSCLE	INSERTION ACTIVITY	POTENTIALS AT REST			MOTOR UNIT POTENTIALS (MUP)				
						Individual MUP			Interference	
			Fib	Pos Waves	Fas	dur (msec)	amp (mV)	% poly-phasic	Pat	amp (mV)
R	Tibialis anterior	N	2+	1+	0	0	0	N	0	0
R	Peroneus longus	N	0	0	0	4	.2	N	1+	.5
R	Gastrocnemius	D	2+	1+	1+	5	.1	Inc	1+	2
L	Vastus Intermedius	D	0	0	0	13	6	N	1+	6
R	First Dorsal Interosseus	D	1+	0	1+	5	10	Inc	1+	12

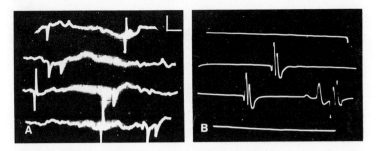

Fig. 5–4. Case 6. Neuronopathy: Wohlfart–Kugelberg–Welander Disease. **A.** Fasciculations and positive waves recorded at rest from the right first dorsal interosseus muscle, coaxial needle electrode. Calibration: 50 μV, 10 msec. **B.** "Giant" polyphasic MUP recorded on minimum voluntary contraction from the right first dorsal interosseus muscle, coaxial electrode. Calibration *(A):* 5 mV, 10 msec/division.

C. *SUMMARY OF FINDINGS AND CLINICAL SIGNIFICANCE.   NSS.* Normal NCV studies. Median distal latency slightly prolonged; the ulnar at upper limits of normal. Prolonged distal latency of right peroneal nerve. *EMG.* Fibrillations and fasciculations noted in several muscles tested. "Giant" MUPs seen in two muscles tested, with increased polyphasic MUPs (Fig. 5–4B).

These findings are compatible with a neuronopathy.

V(b). ENM   (N, brother of patient)
A. *NERVE STIMULATION STUDIES (NSS).*

		LATENCY (msec)				NCV (m/sec)	
		Motor		Sensory			
	Nerve		N		N		N
R	Ulnar	3.2	2.3-3.4			60.6	49-66
L	Peroneal	NR	3.7-6.1			NR	44-58
R	Peroneal	NR	3.7-6.1			NR	44-58
L	Posterior Tibial	6.2	4.2-6.7			50.0	42-55
R	Posterior Tibial	7.0	4.2-6.7			40.8	42-55

B. *ELECTROMYOGRAPHY (EMG).*

L or R	MUSCLE	INSERTION ACTIVITY	POTENTIALS AT REST			MOTOR UNIT POTENTIALS (MUP)				
						Individual MUP			Interference	
			Fib	Pos Waves	Fas	dur (msec)	amp (mV)	% poly-phasic	Pat	amp (mV)
R	Tibialis anterior	N II	0	0	0	8	1	N	1+	1
R	Peroneus longus	D	1+	1+	0	6-7	1.5	N	1+	2
R	Gastrocnemius	N II	1+	0	1+	5	1	N	2+	2
R	Opponens pollicis	D	2+	2+	0	4	5-6	N	1+	6

C. *SUMMARY OF FINDINGS AND CLINICAL SIGNIFICANCE. NSS.*
No response elicited from extensor digitorum brevis muscles on stimulation of either peroneal nerve. The NCV of the right posterior tibial nerve was slightly slowed. The distal latency of the right posterior tibial nerve was slightly prolonged. *EMG.* Fibrillations were seen in most muscles tested, with fasciculations in one. Type II myotonic discharges were noted in two muscles. MUPs relatively normal except for some of high amplitude in the right opponens pollicis muscle.

These findings are compatible with a neuronopathy.

V(c). ENM   (J, brother of patient)
A. *NERVE STIMULATION STUDIES (NSS).*

		LATENCY (msec)				NCV (m/sec)	
		Motor		Sensory			
	Nerve		N		N		N
L	Peroneal	3.5	3.7-6.1			45.7	44-58
R	Peroneal	3.0	3.7-6.1			46.4	44-58

B. *ELECTROMYOGRAPHY (EMG).*

L or R	MUSCLE	INSERTION ACTIVITY	POTENTIALS AT REST			MOTOR UNIT POTENTIALS (MUP)				
						Individual MUP			Interference	
			Fib	Pos Waves	Fas	dur (msec)	amp (mV)	% poly-phasic	Pat	amp (mV)
L	Tibialis anterior	N	It	0	0	7-8	1	Inc	3↑	2
R	Peroneus longus	N	0	0	0	3-5	1	Inc	3↑	1

C. *SUMMARY OF FINDINGS AND CLINICAL SIGNIFICANCE. NSS.*
Normal. *EMG.* Denervation potentials noted in the left tibialis anterior muscle. MUPs highly polyphasic.

These findings are consistent with a denervative process, but in themselves do not indicate a lesion site. If clinically indicated, other muscles should be tested.

VI. COMMENT.   Normal NCV studies were found in the patient. In the first brother, N, stimulation of the peroneal nerves evoked no response from the extensor digitorum brevis muscles although there was contraction of the anterior compartment muscles. This was interpreted as a lack of excitable muscle tissue on the basis of atrophy, rather than evidence of a neuropathy. Although the profound atrophy below the knee raised the question of Charcot–Marie–Tooth Disease (peroneal muscular atrophy), normal NCV studies are against this diagnosis. In the first two brothers, the distal latencies of several nerves were prolonged slightly. This may suggest a distal neuropathy, but can be seen in neuronopathies.

The EMG picture of denervation coupled with abnormally large, long-duration MUPs is compatible with the histologic finding on muscle biopsy of neurogenic atrophy. Together with the familial nature of the condition and the widespread evidence of lower motor neuron involvement on neurologic examination, a diagnosis of chronic proximal spinal muscular atrophy was entertained. The osseous changes are considered an incidental but interesting finding.

In the second brother, J, now in adolesence, there was no clinical evidence of neurologic dysfunction. On EMG, however, denervation was present in the left tibialis anterior muscle. Considering that he shows the same bony changes as his two siblings, it is quite likely that not only the entire family represents an instance of Wohlfart–Kugelberg–Welander Disease, but also that the third brother eventually will become afflicted with similar neurologic involvement.

NEURONOPATHY-NEUROPATHY

Case 7.

PERONEAL MUSCULAR ATROPHY (Charcot-Marie-Tooth Disease)

I. HISTORY.   A 16-year-old white male entered the hospital for evaluation of weakness of the hands and feet. He was born with congenital absence of the right —and possibly the left—clavicle. His mother as well as a brother and sister have this same orthopedic problem. His mother was an only child; her only two siblings were stillborn.

The patient's early motor milestones were perfectly normal. He had attained the 11th grade in school with a B average. At about 5 years of age, his mother noted that he had an unusual gait—a sort of "waddle." When playing he found that he could not run as well as the other children. In the past 3 or 4 years prior to admission, progressive weakness was noted, particularly of the ankles and feet. About 3 or 4 years before the current examination, he found it difficult to control hand movements, particularly when he was cold.

II. PHYSICAL FINDINGS
    A. *General physical examination.* The right clavicle was rudimentary. The right pectoralis group was slightly flat, but strong.
    B. *Neurological examination*
        1. *Mental status and language.* Normal.
        2. *Cranial nerves.* Slight divergent squint of the left eye (strabismus).
        3. *Motor.* Both hands showed weakness of the small muscles, although the opponens pollicis was fairly strong bilaterally. There was a claw hand on both sides, with atrophy in proportion to weakness. No fasciculations were noted. There was a bilateral foot drop of moderate degree and weakness of the gastrocnemius–soleus muscles, more marked on the right than on the left (Fig. 5–5).
        4. *Reflexes.* All muscle-stretch reflexes were present and reduced only in proportion to diminution of power.
        5. *Coordination.* No deficits.
        6. *Sensation.* Normal.

III. LABORATORY DATA.   Lumbar puncture revealed two lymphocytes, a flat colloidal gold curve, and negative serology. The CSF protein was 40 mg%. X ray of the chest was unremarkable except for asymmetry in the configuration of the two clavicles, which was considered developmental and of questionable clinical significance. ENM studies were obtained not only from the patient, but also from his sister and mother.

IV. CLINICAL IMPRESSION.   Peroneal muscular atrophy (Charcot–Marie–Tooth Disease).

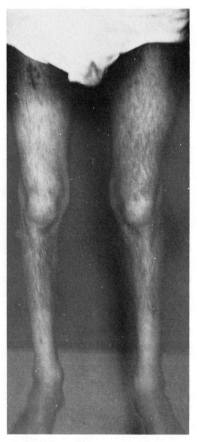

Fig. 5–5. Case 7. Neuronopathy–Neuropathy. Charcot–Marie–Tooth Disease (Peroneal muscular atrophy) Photograph of lower extremities to illustrate atrophy of both legs, especially the left, in contrast to the thighs.

V(a). ENM

A. NERVE STIMULATION STUDIES (NSS).

Nerve		LATENCY (msec)				NCV (m/sec)	
		Motor		Sensory			
			N		N		N
L	Ulnar	5.0	2.3-3.4	4.0	2.1-3.0	41.0	49-66
R	Ulnar	5.2	2.3-3.4	4.6	2.1-3.0	42.0	49-66
L	Peroneal	NR	3.7-6.1			NR	44-58
R	Peroneal	NR	3.7-6.1			NR	44-58

B. ELECTROMYOGRAPHY (EMG).

L or R	MUSCLE	INSERTION ACTIVITY	POTENTIALS AT REST			MOTOR UNIT POTENTIALS (MUP)				
						Individual MUP			Interference	
			Fib	Pos Waves	Fas	dur (msec)	amp (mV)	% poly-phasic	Pat	amp (mV)
R	Deltoid	N	1+	1+	1+	5-8	5	N	1+	5
R	First Dorsal Interosseus	D	2+	1+	1+	5-8	5	N	2+	5
R	Abductor digiti quinti	D	2+	1+	1+	5-8	3	N	2+	5
R	Quadriceps	N	2+	1+	0	5-8	4	N	3+	4
R	Tibialis anterior	D	3+	2+	0	4-6	3	N	0	3
R	Peroneus longus	D	3+	1+	1+	4-6	4	N	0	3
R	Extensor digiti brevis	D	0	0	0	5-8	4	N	0	5
L	Deltoid	N	0	0	0	5-8	4	N	3+	.5
L	First Dorsal Interosseus	D	1+	0	0	5-8	3	N	2+	3
L	Abductor digiti quinti	D	2+	1+	1+	5-8	2	N	2+	3
L	Tibialis anterior	D	3+	1+	1+	5-8	2	N	1+	3
L	Peroneus longus	D	3+	2+	C	5-8	2	N	1+	3
L	Gastrocnemius	N	2+	1+	0	5-8	1	N	1+	2
L	Extensor digiti brevis	D	1+	0	0	5-8	1	N	1+	2

C. SUMMARY OF FINDINGS AND CLINICAL SIGNIFICANCE.   NSS.
Prolonged distal latencies, both sensory and motor, of right and left ulnar nerves. Ulnar NCV slightly slowed bilaterally. No response obtained on stimulating the peroneal nerves on either side. *EMG.* Fibrillations and fasciculations were noted in most muscles tested in all four limbs (Fig. 5–6). MUPs reduced in number and generally increased in amplitude.

These findings are compatible with a lower motor neuron lesion in all four extremities, most likely at the anterior horn cell level. The slightly slow NCV values in the upper limbs can be seen in anterior horn cell syndromes, but no conclusion can be drawn about a neuropathy from the absence of response from the peroneal nerves.

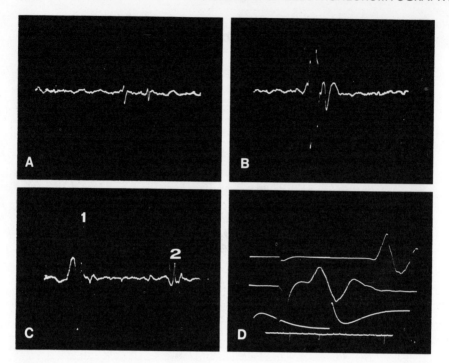

Fig. 5–6. Case 7. Neuronopathy-neuropathy: Peroneal muscular atrophy (Charcot–Marie–Tooth Disease). **A.** Fibrillation potential recorded from right tibialis anterior muscle at rest, coaxial electrode. Calibration: 50 μV, 1 msec/division (see Fig. 5–3A for all calibration signals). **B.** Fasciculation potential recorded from the left tibialis anterior muscle at rest, coaxial needle electrode. Calibration 50 μV, 1 msec/division. **C.** Fibrillation (2) and fasciculation (1) recorded at rest from left tibialis anterior, coaxial electrodes. Calibration 50 μV, 1 msec/division. **D.** Motor NCV of left peroneal nerve: (patient's sister)

	d	t
1	400	15.6
2	45	4.7
3	355	10.9

$$\text{Velocity} = \frac{355}{10.9} = 32.5 \text{ m/sec.}$$

All d and t values are given here and in subsequent calculations in millimeters and milliseconds, respectively; t_3 is obtained by subtraction:

$$V = \frac{d_3 \text{mm}}{t_3 \text{msec}} = \text{m/sec.}$$

V(b). ENM   (Mother of Case 7).
A. *NERVE STIMULATION STUDIES (NSS).*

Nerve	LATENCY (msec)			NCV (m/sec)	
	Motor		Sensory		
		N	N		N
L Ulnar	4.0	2.3-3.4		45.0	49-66
R Ulnar	3.6	2.3-3.4		46.5	49-66

B. *ELECTROMYOGRAPHY (EMG).*

L or R	MUSCLE	INSERTION ACTIVITY	POTENTIALS AT REST			MOTOR UNIT POTENTIALS (MUP)				
						Individual MUP			Interference	
			Fib	Pos Waves	Fas	dur (msec)	amp (mV)	% poly-phasic	Pat	amp (mV)
R	Tibialis anterior	N	1+	0	0	4-6	1-2	N	3+	2.0
L	Tibialis anterior	N	1+	0	0	4-6	1-2	N	3+	2.0

C. *SUMMARY OF FINDINGS AND CLINICAL SIGNIFICANCE.   NSS.*
Slightly slowed NCV of both ulnar nerves. The distal latencies of both ulnar nerves were prolonged slightly. *EMG.* Fibrillations observed in both muscles tested. MUPs were within normal limits.

Compatible with a lower motor neuron lesion of the muscles tested; the slow NCV values suggest a peripheral neuropathy (peroneal muscular atrophy, in view of the findings in the children of this patient).

V(c). ENM   (Sister of Case 7).
A. *NERVE STIMULATION STUDIES (NSS).*

Nerve	LATENCY (msec)			NCV (m/sec)	
	Motor		Sensory		
		N	N		N
L Ulnar	4.1	2.3-3.4		61.0	49-66
R Ulnar	3.9	2.3-3.4		43.5	49-66
L Peroneal	6.2	3.7-6.1		32.5	44-58
R Peroneal	6.5	3.7-6.1		36.0	44-58

B. *ELECTROMYOGRAPHY (EMG).*

L or R	MUSCLE	INSERTION ACTIVITY	POTENTIALS AT REST			MOTOR UNIT POTENTIALS (MUP)				
						Individual MUP			Interference	
			Fib	Pos Waves	Fas	dur (msec)	amp (mV)	% poly-phasic	Pat	amp (mV)
R	First Dorsal Interosseus	N	1+	0	1+	—	—	—	—	—
R	Tibialis anterior	I	2+	1+	1+	—	—	—	—	—
L	First Dorsal Interosseus	N	1+	0	1+	—	—	—	—	—
L	Tibialis anterior	I	2+	1+	1+	—	—	—	—	—

111

C. *SUMMARY OF FINDINGS AND CLINICAL SIGNIFICANCE. NSS.*
NCVs of right ulnar and both peroneal nerves were slowed. Distal latencies of all nerves tested were prolonged slightly. *EMG.* Many fibrillations
and fasciculations were observed in all muscles tested. No MUPs were
produced due to the patient's apparent lack of cooperation.

Compatible with a lower motor neuron lesion in the muscles tested,
specifically a neuropathy of both peroneal nerves. These findings are
consistent with the clinical impression of peroneal muscular atrophy.

VI. COMMENT.   In the patient, the ENM finding of fibrillation potentials in
many muscles points to widespread lower motor neuron disease but has little
precise localizing value. Anterior horn cell involvement is suggested by the
presence of generalized fasciculations, a uniformly poor interference pattern
and MUPs of abnormally high amplitude (enlargement of the motor unit
territory). Although these findings can be seen with lesions other than of the
anterior horn cell, they are typical of the latter. The clinical impression of
peroneal muscular atrophy is not incompatible because this disease may
have a neuronopathic component. On the other hand, slow NCV values almost always are seen in peroneal muscular atrophy. The slightly slow NCV
values for both ulnar nerves suggest peripheral nerve involvement, but can
be seen in some cases of anterior horn cell disease. However, both the
mother and sister of the patient showed slow peroneal NCV values, which
suggests that the same process, i.e., a neuropathy, also is present in the patient. The history and physical findings are concordant with the clinical impression of peroneal muscular atrophy. Anatomic sites of involvement vary
from family to family and this determines what is seen electroneuromyo-
graphically.

NEUROPATHY

Case 8.

PERIPHERAL NEUROPATHY (Diabetic neuropathy)

I. HISTORY.   A 58-year-old white male who had diabetes mellitus for 10 years
came to the neurology clinic. Numbness of the left hand and left half of the face
began 8 years ago. The left foot then became numb and he was told that he had
had a "stroke." A diagnosis of diabetic neuropathy also was made. Since that
time, he complained of occasional sharp pains in the legs and generalized
weakness, both of which became progressively more severe. He took 35 units
of NPH insulin daily.

II. PHYSICAL FINDINGS
   A. *General physical examination.* Unremarkable. Blood pressure and pulse
      were normal.
   B. *Neurologic examination*
      1. *Mental status and language.* No abnormalities.
      2. *Cranial nerves.* There was decreased visual acuity bilaterally, but the
         patient could read the newspaper at arm length.

3. *Motor.* There was distal weakness both in the upper and lower extremities, more marked on the left than on the right.
4. *Reflexes.* The muscle-stretch reflexes were decreased throughout. There were pathologic toe signs on the left.
5. *Coordination.* Gait was broad-based but not ataxic. There were no other deficits.
6. *Sensation.* There was a moderate bilateral stocking loss to pin and cotton, but no deficits to vibration or position sense.

III. LABORATORY DATA.   Laboratory examination revealed normal CBC and urinalysis. FBS, 150 mg%; BUN, 31 mg%. Chest X ray was normal; ECG, nonspecific abnormal (slight S–T segment depression).

IV. CLINICAL IMPRESSION.   1) Peripheral neuropathy associated with diabetes mellitus (diabetic peripheral neuropathy). 2) Residuals of old cerebrovascular accident, right cerebral hemisphere.

V. ENM
   A. *NERVE STIMULATION STUDIES (NSS).*

Nerve		LATENCY (msec)				NCV (m/sec)	
		Motor		Sensory			
			N		N		N
L	*Median*	4.0	2.7-4.2	4.0	2.3-3.2	39.2	48-68
R	*Median*	4.4	2.7-4.2	4.4	2.3-3.2	42.3	48-68
L	*Peroneal*	3.9	3.7-6.1			35.2	44-58
R	*Peroneal*	3.3	3.7-6.1			38.2	44-58

   B. *ELECTROMYOGRAPHY (EMG).*

L or R	MUSCLE	INSERTION ACTIVITY	POTENTIALS AT REST			MOTOR UNIT POTENTIALS (MUP)				
						Individual MUP			Interference	
			Fib	Pos Waves	Fas	dur (msec)	amp (mV)	% polyphasic	Pat	amp (mV)
R	*Tibialis anterior*	N	2+	1+	1+	5-8	1-2	N	2+	2
L	*Tibialis anterior*	N	1+	0	0	5-10	1-2	N	2+	2
R	*Biceps brachii*	N	1+	1+	0	5-10	1-2	N	2+	2

   C. *SUMMARY OF FINDINGS AND CLINICAL SIGNIFICANCE.   NSS.*
   All motor and sensory NCV values are slowed, including upper and lower extremities (Fig. 5–7). *EMG.* Fibrillations noted in all muscles tested; some fasciculations and positive waves also were noted. MUPs within normal limits.
      The ENM findings are those of a diffuse peripheral neuropathy. This is compatible with, but not diagnostic of, the clinical impression of diabetic neuropathy.

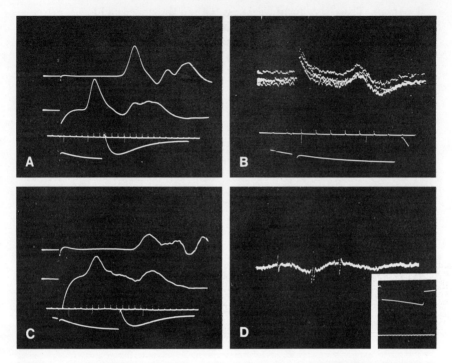

Fig. 5–7. Case 8. Neuropathy: Diabetic peripheral neuropathy. **A.** Motor NCV, left median nerve:

	d	t
1	290	10.1
2	50	40.1
3	240	6.1

$$V = \frac{240}{6.1} = 39.2 \text{ m/sec.}$$

B. Sensory conduction (antidromic), left median nerve: d, 120 mm; t, 4.4 msec.

Latency = 4.4 msec.

$$\text{L.R.} = \frac{120}{4.4} = 27.3 \text{ m/sec}$$

C. Motor NCV, left peroneal nerve:

	d	t
1	355	12.3
2	60	3.9
3	295	8.4

$$V = \frac{295}{8.4} = 35.2 \text{ m/sec.}$$

D. Fibrillation potentials recorded from right tibialis anterior muscle at rest, coaxial needle electrode. Calibration: 50 μV, 1 msec/division.

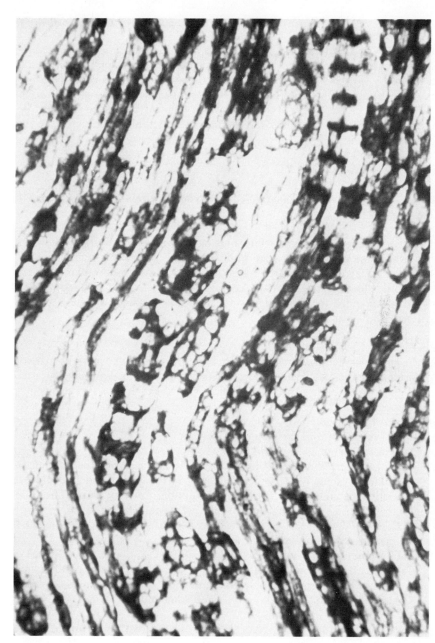

Fig. 5-8. Case 8. Diabetic neuropathy. Section of peripheral nerve root to show Wallerian degeneration. Note the large areas of demyelination and beading. Courtesy of Dr. E. R. Ross. Woelke, ×40.

VI. COMMENT. The slow motor and sensory conduction values are consonant with the clinical impression of a diffuse, bilateral sensorimotor peripheral neuropathy (Fig. 5–8). The relatively normal motor latencies combined with prolonged sensory latencies is the usual circumstance, indicating the earlier vulnerability of the latter. Multiple root involvement cannot be excluded on the basis of the ENM findings, but the history and clinical findings make the correlation secure.

Case 9.

BRACHIAL PLEXUS NEURITIS (Neuralgic Amyotrophy or Syndrome of Parsonage and Turner)*

I. HISTORY. This 50-year-old white male office worker was well until 3 weeks prior to admission when he awoke from sleep with pain in his right shoulder. At noon that day, he was aware of weakness in the arm; within 30 min, he no longer could elevate his right arm. Except for gradual lessening of the pain, these symptoms remained the same for 3 weeks. He had sustained a fracture of the right arm and wrist in childhood.

II. PHYSICAL FINDINGS
  A. *General physical examination.* Examination revealed a cooperative patient in no acute distress. His pulse was regular, and his blood pressure normal. No pain or tenderness was elicited either in the cervical or supraclavicular regions.
  B. *Neurologic examination*
    1. *Mental status and language.* No deficits.
    2. *Cranial nerves.* No deficits.
    3. *Motor.* There was atrophy of the right deltoid, supraspinatus, and infraspinatus muscles. No other focal atrophy was seen. The patient could not abduct the right arm, and external rotation was very weak. The right biceps muscle was relatively strong, but weaker than the left.
    4. *Reflexes.* The muscle-stretch reflexes were brisk and equal throughout. There were no Hoffmann or Babinski signs.
    5. *Coordination.* No deficits.
    6. *Sensation.* There was definite sensory loss to pin prick and cotton touch over the right deltoid muscle at its insertion. No other sensory findings were noted. Vibration and joint sense were intact.

III. LABORATORY DATA. The following were within normal limits: hematocrit, WBC, differential, platelet count, bleeding time, clotting time, ESR, urinalysis, FBS, BUN, serum protein, phosphorous, calcium, alkaline phosphatase, uric acid, and prothrombin time. Spinal puncture revealed an opening pressure equivalent to 185 mm of water with normal dynamics. The CSF contained a total protein of 16 mg% and 90 mg% in the first and third tubes, respectively. Colloidal gold curve was 0111000000. Serology was negative. A glucose tolerance test was normal. X rays of the cervical spine showed

*Plexus latency times were not available at the time of this test.

narrowing of the intervertebral disc space at C5–6 and posterior osteophyte formation at C4–5 and C5–6. Chest x ray was normal. Films of the right elbow showed a loose body in the elbow joint just distal to the radio-humeral articulation, which was thought to represent osteochondritis dessicans. ECG was normal.

Course: He was followed as an outpatient for the next 6 months. Clinical improvement began during the 4th month, heralded by changes in EDX findings at 3 months. Only partial recovery had taken place at the time of the last follow-up visit (5 months).

IV. CLINICAL IMPRESSION.   Brachial plexus neuritis.

V. ENM
   A. ELECTROMYOGRAPHY (EMG).

L or R	MUSCLE	INSERTION ACTIVITY	POTENTIALS AT REST			MOTOR UNIT POTENTIALS (MUP)				
						Individual MUP			Interference	
			Fib	Pos Waves	Fas	dur (msec)	amp (mV)	% poly-phasic	Pat	amp (mV)
R	Deltoid	I	2↑	1↑	0	4-6	.2	N	1↑	.5
R	Supraspinatus	N	2↑	0	0	4-6	.4	N	2↑	.6
R	Infraspinatus	I	2↑	1↑	0	5-8	.4	N	2↑	.5
R	Serratus anterior	N	0	0	0	4-6	1.2	N	3↑	2
R	Biceps brachii	N	0	0	0	4-6	1.2	N	3↑	2
R	Flexor pollicis brevis	N	0	0	0	5-8	1.2	N	3↑	2
L	Deltoid	N	0	0	0	4-6	1.2	N	3↑	2
L	Supraspinatus	N	0	0	0	4-6	1.2	N	3↑	2
L	Biceps brachii	N	0	0	0	4-6	1.2	N	3↑	2
L	Flexor pollicis brevis	N	0	0	0	4-6	1.2	N	3↑	2

   B. SPECIAL STUDIES. S–D curve of the right biceps brachii was normal. S–D curve of the right deltoid muscle showed marked but incomplete denervation (Fig. 5–9)
   C. SUMMARY OF FINDINGS AND CLINCIAL SIGNIFICANCE.   NSS: None performed. EMG: Denervation potentials seen in the right deltoid, supra and infraspinatus muscles, but not in other areas tested. MUPs markedly diminished in number in the right deltoid muscle and somewhat so in the right supra- and infraspinatus muscles. EDX: Normal S–D curve of right biceps brachii, S–D curve of partial denervation in the right deltoid muscle.

   These findings are compatible with partial denervation at the level of the right brachial plexus, upper roots.

VI. COMMENT.   The EMG findings confirmed the presence of a lower motor neuron lesion. Here the localizing value of sampling muscles innervated by different nerves and root levels is evident. Only the deltoid, supraspinatus, and

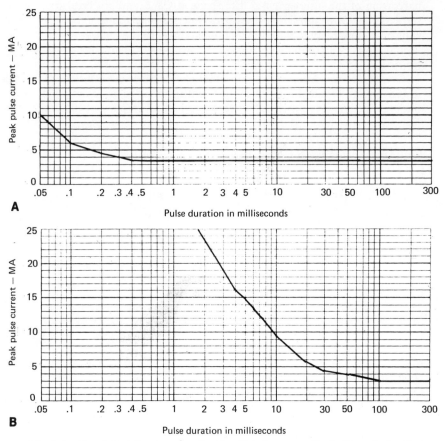

Fig. 5–9. Case 9. Peripheral neuropathy: Brachial plexus neuritis. **A.** Strength duration curve, right biceps brachii muscle, 11/25/64; rheobase, 3.5 ma; chronaxie, 0.08 msec. **B.** Strength duration curve, right deltoid muscle, 11/25/64; rheobase 3.0 ma; chronaxie, 19.0 msec.

infraspinatus muscles on the right side were involved. These muscles are innervated by the 5th and 6th roots of the brachial plexus. The strength–duration curve and EMG of the biceps brachii were normal at the time of first examination, suggesting lack of involvement of the musculocutaneous nerve, originating farther down the plexus, but also from the C5–C6 roots. Thus, assuming brachial plexus involvement, the lesion would seem incomplete. In the case of a root lesion, evidence of denervation would be found in the paraspinal muscles at appropriate root levels.

Serial strength–duration curves traced the course of recovery (Fig. 5–10). The initial curve of the right deltoid was a partial-innervation curve. In the ensuing 5 months, the rheobase initially fell and then rose, typical of denervation followed by reinnervation. This was paralleled by changes in chronaxie, which rose to a maximum 2 months after onset, and then fell toward normal preceding and during clinical recovery. The "improvement" in curve #2, one

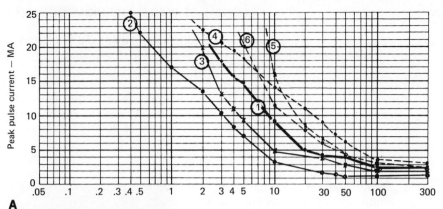

A

Pulse duration in milliseconds

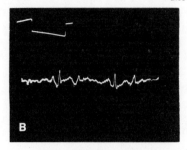

B

Fig. 5–10. Case 9. Peripheral neuropathy: Brachial plexus neuritis. **A.** Composite of 6 strength duration curves taken from right deltoid at various intervals. Rheobase and chronaxie values as shown on chart. **B.** Fibrillation potentials recorded from right deltoid muscle at rest, coaxial electrode. Calibration: 50 μV.

	Date	Rheobase (ma.)	Chronaxie (msec.)
1.	25 November 1964	3.0	19
2.	3 December 1964 (1 week)	1.5	13
3.	24 December 1964 (1 month)	2.0	32
4.	2 February 1965 (2 months)	1.5	125
5.	8 March 1965 (3 months)	2.5	35
6.	28 April 1965 (5 months)	3.0	32

week after the first EDX, was transient, as progressive shift to the right followed in curves #3 through #5. Curve #6 is more normal, but not as much as the initial examination. In this instance, the chronaxie was the most reliable index of reinnervation, because improvement became apparent clinically at 4 months.

The clinical and ENM findings strongly suggest the syndrome of brachial plexus neuritis (neuralgic amyotrophy, the syndrome of Parsonage and Turner).

Case 10.

TARDY ULNAR PALSY

I. HISTORY.   This 40-year-old woman was injured in an automobile accident 18 months prior to examination. While taking a curve too fast, her car turned over and she was unconscious for several minutes. X rays taken at a local emergency room were said to be normal. However, she "wrenched" her right arm. Several months after the accident, she began to complain of numbness and tingling in the fourth and fifth digits of the right hand. She then found it difficult to open car doors and jar lids. Her job involved considerable writing, and she found it difficult to hold a pen. She had no symptoms referable to her neck.

II. PHYSICAL FINDINGS
A. *General physical examination.* The neck was mobile in all directions. On extension of the right arm, there was radial deviation at the elbow. There was a positive Tinel's sign over the ulnar groove of the right elbow.
B. *Neurologic examination*
   1. *Mental status and language.* No deficits.
   2. *Cranial nerves.* No deficits.
   3. *Motor.* There was atrophy and slight weakness of the abductor digiti quinti and interosseous muscles on the right.
   4. *Reflexes.* The muscle-stretch reflexes were brisk and equal.
   5. *Coordination.* No deficits.
   6. *Sensation.* There was minimal loss to pin prick and cotton touch over the fourth and fifth digits of the right hand.

III. LABORATORY DATA.
X ray of the cervical spine revealed minimum degenerative changes; however, no fracture or dislocation was observed. X rays of the elbows were normal.

IV. CLINICAL IMPRESSION.
Tardy ulnar palsy.

V. ENM
A. *NERVE STIMULATION STUDIES (NSS).*

	Nerve	LATENCY (msec)				NCV (m/sec)	
		Motor		Sensory			
			N		N		N
R	Ulnar elbow-wrist	2.6	2.3-3.4			50.0	49-66
R	Ulnar across elbow					44.9	49-66
R	Ulnar axilla - elbow					55.0	50-74
L	Ulnar elbow-wrist	2.9	2.3-3.4			53.0	49-66
L	Ulnar across elbow					54.5	49-66
L	Ulnar axilla - elbow					56.0	50-74

B. *ELECTROMYOGRAPHY (EMG).*

L or R	MUSCLE	INSERTION ACTIVITY	POTENTIALS AT REST			MOTOR UNIT POTENTIALS (MUP)				
						Individual MUP			Interference	
			Fib	Pos Waves	Fas	dur (msec)	amp (mV)	% poly-phasic	Pat	amp (mV)
R	First Dorsal Interosseus	I	3+	2+	1+	5-7	1.5	N	3+	1.5
R	Abductor digiti V	I	1+	0	0	5-7	2.0	N	3+	4
R	Triceps	N	0	0	0	5-7	5-2	N	3+	2

C. *SUMMARY OF FINDINGS AND CLINICAL SIGNIFICANCE.* *NSS:* Slowed ulnar NCV across the elbow on the right. *EMG:* Fibrillations and fasciculations noted in the right first dorsal interosseus and abductor digiti quinti muscles.

These findings are compatible with a partial segmental ulnar nerve lesion at the right elbow.

VI. COMMENT. Electromyography revealed denervation potentials in the small hand muscles supplied by the ulnar nerve. The right triceps was normal, however, so that evidence of clinical or ENM involvement was not found above the elbow. Further study of proximal muscles, such as the paraspinal group, might have been helpful. This is important if a lesion *at* the elbow is suspected. Nerve conduction velocity studies confirmed this by showing a normal ulnar NCV on the left, and above the right elbow. However, at this level (across the elbow) on the right side, NCV was slowed.

On the basis of these findings, the right ulnar nerve was transplanted to the anterior surface of the elbow. Clinical improvement followed.

Case 11.

CARPAL TUNNEL SYNDROME

I. HISTORY. This 40-year-old right-handed white female was referred because of "numbness" (paresthesias) of the left hand. She was well until 19 years prior to examination, when these symptoms became apparent while knitting. The sensation of numbness would spread to the elbow and last as long as the patient was working, but would disappear a few minutes after she stopped. Seven years later, she developed numbness in both hands related to such activities as playing golf. Five years before examination, she developed pain in both arms which became constant 2 years later. It was unrelated to effort and became worse at night. Touching objects produced an "electric" sensation in her fingers.

An "aberrant thyroid" was removed surgically in 1950, followed by radioactive iodine treatment. She had been taking thyroid extract ever since. On two occasions, she fainted; an EEG revealed "mild epilepsy." A glucose tolerance test was said to show "hypoglycemia." At the time of consultation, she was taking thyroid extract, 3 gr daily; chlorthiazide, 250 mg bid; and dextroamphetamine, 5 mg daily.

II. PHYSICAL FINDINGS
   A. *General physical examination.* Blood pressure was 138/90. Her face was plethoric with puffy cheeks and a "buffalo hump." Adson's maneuver was positive on extreme hyperabduction of each arm. During this procedure, some numbness of the right fifth finger of the right hand was produced. When a blood pressure cuff around the arm was inflated to above systolic blood pressure, the right fifth finger became more numb than the other fingers. Tinel's sign was negative.
   B. *Neurologic examination*
      1. *Mental status and language.* Normal.
      2. *Cranial nerves.* Slight exophthalmos, otherwise normal.

3. *Motor.* Gait and station were normal, including heel, toe, and tandem walking. There was minimal weakness of the right first dorsal interosseous muscle, flexor carpi ulnaris, and abductor digiti quinti muscles on the right. These minimal findings were thought to be due to guarding of the hand.
4. *Reflexes.* The muscle-stretch reflexes were brisk and equal, and the plantar responses were flexor.
5. *Coordination.* No deficits.
6. *Sensation.* Normal.

III. LABORATORY DATA.   Cervical spine X ray revealed some narrowing of the third and fourth cervical interspaces posteriorly, with some spurring, particularly in the intervertebral foramina of the third interspace.

IV. CLINICAL IMPRESSION.   Carpal tunnel syndrome? Scalenus Anticus syndrome?

V. ENM
   A. *NERVE STIMULATION STUDIES (NSS).*

		LATENCY (msec)				NCV (m/sec)	
		Motor		Sensory			
	Nerve		N		N		N
L	Ulnar	2.7	2.3-3.4			57.0	49-66
R	Ulnar	3.0	2.3-3.4	3.0	2.1-3.0	56.0	49-66
L	Median	4.2	2.7-4.2			48.0	48-68
R	Median	6.0	2.7-4.2	5.0	2.3-3.2	51.0	48-68

   B. *ELECTROMYOGRAPHY (EMG).*

L or R	MUSCLE	INSERTION ACTIVITY	POTENTIALS AT REST			MOTOR UNIT POTENTIALS (MUP)				
						Individual MUP			Interference	
			Fib	Pos Waves	Fas	dur (msec)	amp (mV)	% poly-phasic	Pat	amp (mV)
R	Triceps brachii	N	0	0	0	5-8	1-2	N	3+	2
L	Triceps brachii	N	0	0	0	5-8	1-2	N	3+	2
L	Brachiorodialis	N	0	0	0	5-8	1-2	N	3+	2
R	First dorsal interosseus	N	0	0	0	5-8	1-2	N	3+	2
L	First dorsal interosseus	N	0	0	0	5-8	1-2	N	3+	2
R	Abductor digiti V	N	0	0	0	6-8	1-2	N	3+	2
L	Abductor digiti V	N	0	0	0	5-8	1-2	N	3+	2
R	Opponens pollicis	N	0	0	0	5-8	1-2	N	3+	2

C. *SUMMARY OF FINDINGS AND CLINICAL SIGNIFICANCE. NSS.*
Motor and sensory distal latencies of the right median nerve were slowed
(Fig. 5–11A); otherwise, normal NCV and latency studies (Fig. 5–11B).
EMG. Within normal limits.

These findings are compatible with the clinical impression of a carpal
tunnel syndrome on the right.

VI. COMMENT. See case 12.

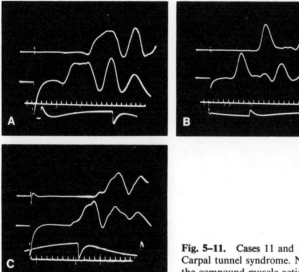

Fig. 5–11. Cases 11 and 12. Compression neuropathy:
Carpal tunnel syndrome. Note the abnormal contour of
the compound muscle action potentials.

A. Case 11, Motor NCV, right nedian nerve:

	d	t
1	290	10.7
2	50	6.0
3	240	4.7

Latency = 6.0 msec.

$$V = \frac{240}{4.7} = 51.1 \text{ m/sec.}$$

B. Case 11, Motor NCV left median nerve:

	d	t
1	295	9.2
2	55	4.2
3	240	5.0

Latency = 4.2 msec.

$$V = \frac{240}{5.0} = 48.0 \text{ m/sec.}$$

C. Case 12, Motor NCV right median nerve:

	d	t
1	285	12.2
2	55	7.3
3	230	4.9

Latency = 7.3 msec.

$$V = \frac{230}{4.9} = 47.0 \text{ m/sec.}$$

Case 12.

CARPAL TUNNEL SYNDROME

I. HISTORY.   A 55-year-old white female described her complaints, present for the past 10 years, as tingling and paresthesias of her right hand, brought on by knitting, writing, and other tasks requiring use of her hand. The thumb and first three fingers were involved, including the medial aspect of the fourth finger. She was employed as a comptroller prior to evaluation, and was right-handed.

Following an automobile accident 13 months prior to evaluation, pain began in the right shoulder area. Surgery performed on the shoulder relieved some of the pain, but the hand then became significantly more paresthetic and painful. The pain was worse at night and often prevented sleep.

The patient had similar complaints referable to the opposite hand, but not as severe as the right. The hands were neither weak nor clumsy. Her general medical health had been good.

II. PHYSICAL FINDINGS
   A. *General physical examination.* Unremarkable. Blood pressure 155/85.
   B. *Neurologic examination*
      1. *Mental status and language.* No deficits.
      2. *Cranial nerves.* No deficits.
      3. *Motor.* There was questionable atrophy of the right abductor pollicis brevis but no other motor loss was noted in the upper limbs; there was no atrophy and there were no fasciculations. Tinel's sign was positive over the right carpal tunnel. Inflation of a blood pressure cuff around the arm markedly increased the patient's symptoms.
      4. *Reflexes.* The muscle-stretch reflexes were symmetrical throughout.
      5. *Coordination.* No deficits.
      6. *Sensation.* There was hypesthesia and hypalgesia over the second and third fingers of the right hand on the palmar surface and over half of the fourth finger. This sensory loss extended partway into the palm.

IV. CLINICAL IMPRESSION.   Carpal tunnel syndrome.

V. ENM
   A. *NERVE STIMULATION STUDIES (NSS).*

	Nerve	LATENCY (msec)				NCV (m/sec)	
		Motor		Sensory			
			N		N		N
L	Ulnar	2.2	2.3-3.4			53.3	49-66
R	Ulnar	2.2	2.3-3.4			54.5	49-66
L	Median	4.5	2.7-4.2	3.0	2.3-3.2	48.0	48-68
R	Median	7.3	2.7-4.4	5.4	2.3-3.2	47.0	48-68

B. *ELECTROMYOGRAPHY (EMG)*.

L or R	MUSCLE	INSERTION ACTIVITY	POTENTIALS AT REST			MOTOR UNIT POTENTIALS (MUP)				
						Individual MUP			Interference	
			Fib	Pos Waves	Fas	dur (msec)	amp (mV)	% poly-phasic	Pat	amp (mV)
R	Opponens pollicis	N	1+	0	0	5-8	1:2	N	.3+	2
L	Opponens pollicis	N	0	0	0	5-8	1:2	N	3+	2

C. *SUMMARY OF FINDINGS AND CLINICAL SIGNIFICANCE.   NSS.*
NCV values for ulnar nerves are normal; those of median nerves, at lower
limits of normal (Fig. 5-11C). The motor and sensory distal latencies are
at the upper limits of normal on the left and prolonged on the right. *EMG.*
a few fibrillations noted in right thenar muscle.

These findings are compatible with a right carpal tunnel syndrome.

VI. COMMENT.   (Cases 11 and 12) The prolonged latency across the right
carpal tunnel in Case 11 is compatible with the clinical impression of carpal
tunnel syndrome, with the left latency at the upper limits of normal. In some
cases of carpal tunnel syndrome, the distal median nerve motor latency is
normal and only the sensory latency is prolonged. In rare instances, both can
be normal. Likewise the normal EMG findings do not exclude this diagnosis.
In view of the neurologic history and findings, which are at best atypical for
an entrapment neuropathy, the electromyographer was wise in his cautious
statement, "compatible with a diagnosis of carpal tunnel syndrome." It then
becomes the clinician's responsibility to decide whether the marginal latency
values are evidence enough to justify the impression, or whether further search
should be made for other pathology.

Case 12 is more typical of carpal tunnel syndrome from both the clinical
and ENM standpoints. Although questionable atrophy was apparent, the
distribution of the pain, paresthesias, sensory loss, and a positive Tinel's sign
are all consonant with a carpal tunnel syndrome. The latency value of 7.3 msec
across the right carpal tunnel confirms the diagnosis. These findings emphasize
the value of ENM in early diagnosis, and help to exclude a more proximal root
lesion.

NEUROPATHY (ROOT SYNDROME)

Case 13.

HERNIATED NUCLEUS PULPOSUS

I. HISTORY.   One month prior to examination, a 44-year-old male was unload-
ing a truck of canteloupe when he twisted his back. Since that time, he experienced continual back and leg pain. He described it as radiating down both
legs to the big toes on each foot. A sharp pain was brought on by coughing,
laughing, or sneezing. He also experienced "tingling" in the feet. On rare

occasions, he felt that his right leg was weak because the knee would buckle. Extension of the back was painful. He had been unable to work after the accident.

II. PHYSICAL FINDINGS
    A. *General physical examination.* There was tenderness to palpation to the right of the L4–L5 spinous processes.
    B. *Neurologic examination*
        1. *Mental status and language.* No deficits.
        2. *Cranial nerves.* No deficits.
        3. *Motor.* The Kernig and straight-leg-raising tests evoked pain and reflex spasm on the right, but not on the left. There was no clonus or atrophy. No motor deficits were observed.
        4. *Reflexes.* The right-ankle jerk was diminished compared to the left, but the knee jerks were equal. No pathologic reflexes were illicited.
        5. *Coordination.* No deficits.
        6. *Sensation.* There was hypesthesia and hypalgesia along the lateral border of the right leg and foot.

III. LABORATORY DATA. A lumbar myelogram (Fig. 5–12A) revealed slight assymetry of the nerve root sleeves at the L4–L5 level. A cross-table view revealed a slight impression of the anterior aspect of the spinal canal at the L4–L5 level. Spinal fluid protein was at the upper limits of normal, 45 mg%; no cells were noted. The remainder of the spinal fluid examination was within normal limits.

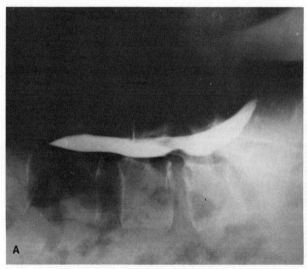
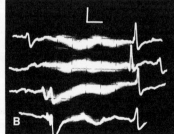

Fig. 5–12. Case 13. Neuropathy. Herniated nucleus pulposus. **A.** Lumbar myelogram, cross-table lateral view. Filling defect at L4–L5 compatible with a herniated disc. Courtesy of Dr. E. Palacios. **B.** Fibrillations recorded from the left tibialis anterior at rest; coaxial needle electrode. Calibration: 50 μV, 5 msec.

IV. CLINICAL IMPRESSION. Herniated nucleus pulposus at L4–L5, right.

V. ENM

  A. *NERVE STIMULATION STUDIES (NSS).*

Nerve		LATENCY (msec)				NCV (m/sec)	
		Motor		Sensory			
			N		N		N
L	Peroneal	4.2	3.7-6.1			54.8	44-58
R	Peroneal	4.8	3.7-6.1			51.5	44-58
L	Posterior Tibial	6.0	4.2-6.7			60.0	42-55
R	Posterior Tibial	5.5	4.2-6.7			46.3	42-55

  B. *ELECTROMYOGRAPHY (EMG).*

L or R	MUSCLE	INSERTION ACTIVITY	POTENTIALS AT REST			MOTOR UNIT POTENTIALS (MUP)				
						Individual MUP			Interference	
			Fib	Pos Waves	Fas	dur (msec)	amp (mV)	% poly-phasic	Pat	amp (mV)
R	Tibialis anterior	I	2+	1+	0	5	.5-1.5	Inc	2+	4
R	Gastrocnemius	N	1+	0	0	6	.5-1.5	N	2+	2
R	Peroneus longus	N	1+	0	0	5-6	.5-1.5	N	3+	2
L	Tibialis anterior	I	3+	2+	0	3-5	.4	Inc	2+	1.5
R	Vastus intermedius	N	0	0	0	5-8	1-1.5	N	3+	2
L	Vastus intermedius	N	0	0	0	5-8	1.5-2.0	N	3+	2

  C. *SUMMARY OF FINDINGS AND CLINICAL SIGNIFICANCE.* *NSS.* Normal NCV values; but note difference between right and left posterior tibial nerves. *EMG.* denervation potentials present in several muscles but especially in both tibialis anterior muscles (Fig. 5–12B). MUPs relatively normal except for increased numbers of polyphasic MUPs in some areas.

  Bilateral denervation suggesting involvement of the root segments L4–L5.

VI. COMMENT. Motor NCVs in both legs were normal. This is not uncommon in the presence of a herniated nucleus pulposus at a given level, because multiple root involvement must be present before significant slowing of the motor NCV occurs in the fastest fibers. On the other hand, the posterior tibial NCV on the left was slower than the right, which correlates with the clinically involved side. Fibrillations noted in the tibialis anterior muscles on both sides suggested the presence of denervation at the L4–L5 level. It is also important that muscles above the knees failed to reveal evidence of denervation; only the L4–L5 segment was involved.

  In cases of suspect root involvement, it is important to study the paraspinal muscles at levels that correspond to the clinically suspect site of involvement.

Unfortunately, this was not done in the present case, so that this information is not available. When searching for denervation potentials in the paraspinal muscles, it is most important to secure complete relaxation, because these muscles tend to be tonically active and the persistant MUPs make their recognition difficult.

Surgery was performed. A herniated nucleus pulposus was found in the L4–L5 level and removed. The patient made an uneventful recovery and his symptoms were relieved.

Case 14.

CERVICAL SPONDYLOSIS

I. HISTORY.   A 54-year-old white male was admitted to the hospital because of pain and numbness in the hands for the past year. These symptoms had been progressive during the past 6 months together with impaired coordination and weakness of the hands.

II. PHYSICAL FINDINGS
  A. *General physical examination.* There was definite limitation of neck motion in all 6 directions, especially extension of the neck.
  B. *Neurologic examination.*
    1. *Mental status and language.* No deficits.
    2. *Cranial nerves.* No deficits.
    3. *Motor.* Gait was normal, including toe and heel walking and tandem gait. There was slight atrophy of the thenar and hypothenar eminences but no fasciculations were observed. These muscles were correspondingly weak. Aside from this, there were no motor deficits.
    4. *Reflexes.* The knee and ankle jerks were symmetrically brisk, but there was no clonus and there were no Babinski signs.
    5. *Coordination.* Coordination of the hands was impaired markedly; pseudoathetotic movements due to sensory loss were observed. He could perform very few skilled movements with his hands.
    6. *Sensation.* There was profound loss of vibration and position sense in the upper extremities, with minimal hypesthesia and hypalgesia in a glove distribution to the wrists on both sides.

III. LABORATORY DATA.   X rays of the neck revealed marked narrowing of the intervertebral joint spaces between C4–C5, with spur formation projecting anteriorly and posteriorly. A cervical myelogram (Fig. 5–13A) showed compression (filling defects) of the column of contrast medium at this level, particularly on the cross-table view. The CSF protein was 85 mg%. Additional X rays, including upper GI, lower GI, and IVP, were all within normal limits. Routine CBC, urinalysis, and chest X ray were all normal. Acid phosphatase was within normal limits (7 units).

IV. CLINICAL IMPRESSION.   Cervical spondylosis.

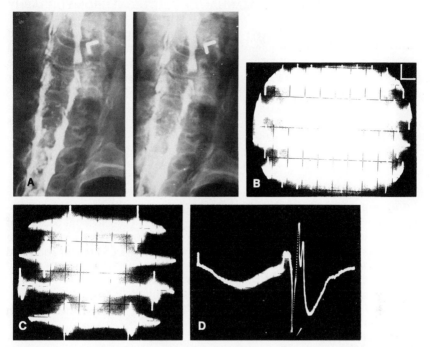

Fig. 5–13. Neuropathy: Case 14. Cervical spondylosis. **A.** Cervical myelogram. Slight widening of the cervical spinal cord; filling defects noted at C4–C5 and root sleeve asymmetries at lower levels. **B.** Myotonic discharge type II recorded at rest from the left deltoid muscle, evoked by needle insertion in the absence of clinical myotonia, coaxial electrode. Note lack of decrescendo pattern (sustained discharge). Calibration: 1 mV, 50 msec (frequency of discharge = 20/sec). The four traces are sequentially displayed. **C.** Same as A, but calibration = 10 msec. Note repetitive polyphasic units. **D.** Motor latency to left deltoid muscle; recording needle electrode 16 cm distal to stimulation site over brachial plexus (Erb's point). Calibration: 1 mV, 2 msec. Latency = 11.2 msec. X rays courtesy of Dr. E. Palacios.

V. ENM

A. *NERVE STIMULATION STUDIES (NSS).*

	Nerve	LATENCY (msec)				NCV (m/sec)	
		Motor		Sensory			
			N		N		N
L	Ulnar	4.0	2.3-3.4			47.0	49-66
R	Ulnar	3.5	2.3-3.4			45.0	49-66
L	Median	5.6	2.7-4.2			53.3	48-68
R	Median	4.0	2.7-4.2			44.5	48-68
L	Peroneal	5.2	3.7-6.1			48.9	44-58
R	Peroneal	4.8	3.7-6.1			49.3	44-58
R	Posterior Tibial	5.2	4.2-6.7			56.8	42-55
L	Axillary	11.2	<4.5 at 16 cm				

129

B. *ELECTROMYOGRAPHY (EMG).*

L or R	MUSCLE	INSERTION ACTIVITY	POTENTIALS AT REST			MOTOR UNIT POTENTIALS (MUP)				
						Individual MUP			Interference	
			Fib	Pos Waves	Fas	dur (msec)	amp (mV)	% poly-phasic	Pat	amp (mV)
L	First dorsal interosseus	N	3+	1+	2+	4-5	2	N	2+	2
L	Deltoid	M II	0	0	0	5	2	N	2+	2
R	Opponens pollicis	N	2+	1+	1+	5-6	1-2	Inc	2+	1
R	Biceps brachii	N	2+	1+	0	5-6	2	N	2+	1.5

C. *SUMMARY OF FINDINGS AND CLINICAL SIGNIFICANCE.* *NSS:* mild slowing of NCVs in three of four nerves in the upper limbs. The terminal latencies of the left median and both ulnar nerves were prolonged, as was the latency time of the left axillary nerve to the left deltoid muscle (Figs. 5–13B, C, and D). *EMG.* Denervation potentials noted in the small hand muscles and the right biceps brachii; fasciculations were noted in several areas. MUPs relatively normal.

These findings are compatible with a lower motor neuron lesion in both upper extremities, C5–T1, most severe in the C7–T1 segments. The slow NCV values suggest either peripheral nerve or multiple root involvement; the latter correlates with the clinical impression of cervical spondylosis.

VI. COMMENT. The EMG findings revealed evidence of denervation in most muscles tested. In addition, type II myotonic discharges were elicited on needle insertion, a finding which, although not diagnostic of, can be seen with root involvement. The parameters of the MUPs were all relatively normal, which speaks against anterior horn cell involvement. Nerve conduction velocity studies revealed slight slowing in three of the four nerves in the upper extremities. Although this also is compatible with a peripheral neuropathy, clinical correlation with multiple root involvement was considered a reasonable cause, especially in view of the prolonged latency value to the left deltoid, a proximal muscle.

An anterior cervical fusion was performed, using a bone graft from the right hip. Following surgery, the patient made a fairly uneventful recovery, but was not relieved of symptoms entirely. He continued to complain of some pain and tingling in the fingers but there was definite improvement in the neurologic picture.

NEUROPATHY

Case 15.

ACUTE ASCENDING POLYRADICULONEURITIS (Guillain–Barré Syndrome)

I. HISTORY. A 24-year-old male dental student was brought to the hospital because of increasing weakness. He had been well until 1 month previously, when he developed diarrhea, fever, and "stomach flu." He then began to feel increasingly ill, with weakness of the lower extremities on climbing stairs, numbness and tingling of the feet and hands, and a "lump in his throat." Four days later, swallowing and speaking became difficult. Weakness of the upper limbs was followed a few days later by a similar loss of function of the right side of the face. These progressive symptoms prompted admission to the hospital.

II. PHYSICAL FINDINGS
    A. *General physical examination.* No deficits.
    B. *Neurologic examination*
        1. *Mental status and language.* Speech was nasal and articulation was difficult.
        2. *Cranial nerves.* There was incomplete paralysis of the entire right side of the face, including the forehead. The uvula deviated to the left and the anterior neck muscles were weak.
        3. *Motor.* Gait was quite unsteady, and he was unable to squat and then stand. Toe and heel walking also were weak. Proximal muscle groups of all four extremities were quite weak but there was no atrophy.
        4. *Reflexes.* The muscle-stretch reflexes were absent throughout, even with reinforcement. The abdominal reflexes were brisk on both sides. There were no meningeal signs.
        5. *Coordination.* Limited only by weakness.
        6. *Sensation.* There was slight sensory impairment over the legs to light touch but not to pin prick. Vibration was slightly diminished at both ankles.

III. LABORATORY DATA. Urinalysis, normal; Hgb, 18 mg %; Hct, 53%; WBC, 6400; ESR, 1 mm /hour; FBS, 98 mg %; phosphorus and alkaline phosphatase, normal; serum glutamic oxalacetic transaminase, 20 units; urine porphobilinogen, negative; heterophile antibody titer, 1:7; cold agglutinins, 1:64. Spinal fluid findings: total protein, 170 mg %; electrophoresis: alpha globulin, 28%; beta, 12%; alpha, 1 and alpha 2, 21%; albumin, 39%; spinal fluid glucose, 65 mg %; 2 lymphocytes; flat colloidal gold curve. Culture of the spinal fluid for bacteria and fungi was negative, as were direct smears for bacteria, acid-fast bacilli, and india ink preparations. An electroencephalogram was normal as were X rays of the chest and skull.

IV. CLINICAL IMPRESSION. Guillain–Barré Syndrome (acute ascending polyradiculoneuritis).

V. ENM

A. *NERVE STIMULATION STUDIES (NSS).*

	Nerve	LATENCY (msec)				NCV (m/sec)	
		Motor		Sensory			
			N		N		N
R	ulnar	3.6	2.3-3.4			47.2	49-66
L	Median	8.6	2.7-4.2			44.5	48-68
R	Median	10.7	2.7-4.2			37.0	48-68
R	Peroneal	9.2	3.7-6.1			45.0	44-58
L	Posterior Tibial	11.7	4.2-6.7			35.8	42-55

B. *ELECTROMYOGRAPHY (EMG).*

L or R	MUSCLE	INSERTION ACTIVITY	POTENTIALS AT REST			MOTOR UNIT POTENTIALS (MUP)				
						Individual MUP			Interference	
			Fib	Pos Waves	Fas	dur (msec)	amp (mV)	% poly-phasic	Pat	amp (mV)
L	Deltoid	D	0	0	0	5-8	1-2	Inc	2+	2
R	First dorsal interosseus	D	+	0	0	5-8	1-2	Inc	2+	2
L	Tibialis anterior	D	0	0	0	5-8	1-2	Inc	2+	2
R	Gastrocnemius	D	0	0	0	5-8	1-2	Inc	2+	2

C. *SUMMARY OF FINDINGS AND CLINICAL SIGNIFICANCE. NSS.*
Prolonged terminal latencies in all nerves tested (Figs. 5–14C and D). NCV values slowed to a greater or lesser degree in all nerves tested except the right peroneal. *EMG.* A few fibrillations were noted in the right first dorsal interosseus muscle (Figs. 5–14A and B); interference pattern decreased in all muscles tested with increased numbers of polyphasic MUPs.

The ENM findings are consistent with a diffuse peripheral neuropathy involving all extremities. These findings are compatible with the clinical impression of polyradiculo-neuropathy (Guillain–Barré syndrome).

VI. COMMENT.
The ENM findings point to a disease of the multiple peripheral nerves in all four extremities. The slow NCVs, prolonged distal latencies, absence of fasciculations, and normal MUP parameters suggest peripheral nerve involvement rather than anterior horn cell. Because the test was done early in the disease, only minimal fibrillation was noted. EMG evaluation of paraspinal muscles may have helped clarify the site of lesion.

The ENM correlation with the history, examination and laboratory data are compatible with the clinical diagnosis of Guillain–Barré syndrome. The ENM findings in this disorder vary with the severity of the disorder and the stage of the disease at the time of examination.

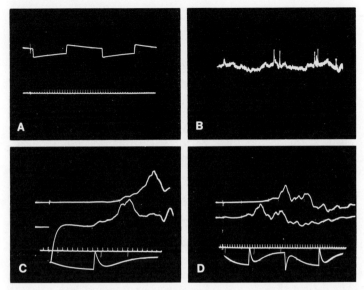

Fig. 5–14.   Case 15. Acute ascending polyradiculoneuritis (Guillain–Barré Syndrome) **A.**
Calibration signal for B. **B.** Muscle at rest; right 1st dorsal interosseus, monopolar recording.
Calibration: (A) 50 μV, 1 msec/division. **C.** Motor NCV, left median nerve (note decreased
amplitude and prolonged duration of the compound muscle action potential):

	d	t
1	300	14.1
2	55	8.6
3	245	5.5

$$V = \frac{245}{5.5} = 44.5 \text{ m/sec.}$$

D. Motor NCV, left posterior tibial nerve:

	d	t
1	440	22.2
2	65	11.7
3	375	10.5

$$V = \frac{375}{10.5} = 35.8 \text{ m/sec.}$$

NEUROMYAL JUNCTION

Case 16.

MYASTHENIA GRAVIS

I. HISTORY.   A 36-year-old right-handed white female gave a 6 year history of myasthenia gravis, which began with fatigue of lip movement. The weakness spread to other muscles of the lower face and pharynx and finally to the legs, particularly the left. A thymectomy was performed without definite improvement. In 5 years, she lost 80 pounds. The illness rapidly progressed until she could swallow only with difficulty.

II. PHYSICAL FINDINGS
  A. *General physical examination.* Unremarkable.
  B. *Neurologic examination*
     1. *Mental status and language.* No deficits.
     2. *Cranial nerves.* Her voice was nasal, the protruded tongue tremulous, and her facies myopathic. She could not pucker or whistle.
     3. *Motor.* The patient climbed up on her legs when standing from a supine or sitting position (Gower's sign). The proximal muscles were all weak, but there was no atrophy.
     4. *Reflexes.* The plantar responses were flexor and abdominal reflexes were diminished. The muscle-stretch reflexes were uniformly hypoactive.
     5. *Coordination.* No deficits.
     6. *Sensation.* Normal.

III. LABORATORY DATA.   Examination of the blood, electrolytes, and serology were all within normal limits. An electroencephalogram showed very minimal right temporal slowing. Intravenous edrophonium was given with minimal improvement, but side effects resulted thereafter.

   She was placed on ambenonium, 15–20 mg q4h with ephedrine, 25 mg tid. She improved markedly on this regimen.

IV. CLINICAL IMPRESSION.   Myasthenia gravis.

V. ENM
  A. *NERVE STIMULATION STUDIES (NSS).*

		LATENCY (msec)			NCV (m/sec)	
		Motor		Sensory		
	Nerve		N		N		N
L	Posterior Tibial	4.2	4.2-6.7			41.5	42-55

B. *ELECTROMYOGRAPHY (EMG).*

L or R	MUSCLE	INSERTION ACTIVITY	POTENTIALS AT REST			MOTOR UNIT POTENTIALS (MUP)				
						Individual MUP			Interference	
			Fib	Pos Waves	Fas	dur (msec)	amp (mV)	% poly-phasic	Pat	amp (mV)
L	Vastus Medialis	D	0	0	0	4·8	1·2	N	2+	2
L	Rectus Femoris	D	0	0	0	4·8	1·2	N	2+	2
L	Vastus Lateralis	D	0	0	0	4·8	1·2	N	2+	2
L	Biceps Femoris	N	0	0	0	4·8	1·2	N	3+	2

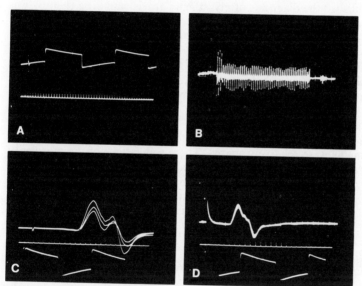

Fig. 5–15. Cases 16 and 17. Myasthenia Gravis. **A.** Calibration signal for B, 1 mV, 1 msec/div. **B.** Case 16. Repetitive stimulation of right median nerve at the wrist (Method II) at 30 stimuli/sec. **C.** Case 17. Repetitive stimulation of the right median nerve at the elbow (Method I) using 3/sec. stimuli before administration of edrophonium. *D* same as C, taken shortly thereafter; repetitive stimulation at the wrist to illustrate reversal of neuromuscular fatigability (amplitude falloff) produced by intravenous administration of edrophonium.

C. *SPECIAL STUDIES.*   Repetitive stimulation of the right median nerve (Figs. 5–15A and B) at the wrist (recording from the thenar muscles) with stimuli of 30/sec produced a typical myasthenic response (50% decline of the evoked response).

D. *SUMMARY OF FINDINGS AND CLINICAL SIGNIFICANCE. NSS.* Essentially normal conduction velocity of the nerve tested. Repetitive stimulation produced a typical myasthenic response. *EMG.* No denervation potentials were observed. MUP normal except reduced interference pattern observed in three of four muscles tested.

These findings are compatible with the clinical impression of myasthenia gravis.

VI. COMMENT.   See Case 17.

Case 17.

MYASTHENIA GRAVIS

I. HISTORY.   A 73-year-old physician described the onset of his disease 12 months prior to admission as slurring of speech, difficulty swallowing, ptosis of the eyelids, and generalized muscular weakness. Three months later, a neostigmine test established the diagnosis of myasthenia gravis, and drug therapy was instituted (pyridostigmine and atropine).

II. PHYSICAL FINDINGS
A. *General physical examination.* There was generalized lymphadenopathy in the occipital, cervical, submandibular, axillary, and inguinal regions. The tip of the spleen was just palpable. There was pitting edema of both ankles.
B. *Neurologic examination*
  1. *Mental status and language.* Normal.
  2. *Cranial nerves.* There was bilateral ptosis but the extraocular muscle movements were relatively spared. There was fatigue of the muscles of mastication and swallowing, with nasal speech.
  3. *Motor.* Rapid fatigue was evident during any muscular activity and this was especially obvious on repetitive hand grasp. His gait was unsteady, probably due to weakness. Intravenous edrophonium rapidly reversed the weakness.
  4. *Reflexes.* Within normal limits.
  5. *Coordination.* No deficits.
  6. *Sensation.* No deficits.

III. LABORATORY DATA.   Total protein, 6.3 mg%; albumin, 3.3 mg %; globulin, 3.0 mg %. ECG revealed evidence of a recent myocardial infarction. Chest X ray revealed a tortuous aorta, but was otherwise normal. Lymph node biopsy revealed a histologic pattern of lymphosarcoma, small-cell type. *HOSPITAL COURSE.* The patient had a stormy course, almost dying from crises on several occasions. X ray therapy was given to the right groin (2300 rad), right axilla (2300 rad), and left groin (2500 rad). Whether coincidental, or as a result of therapy, there was considerable improvement following irradiation.

IV. CLINICAL IMPRESSION.   1) Myasthenia gravis associated with 2) lymphosarcoma, small cell type; 3) myocardial infarction.

V. ENM
A. *SPECIAL STUDIES.* Repetitive stimulation: 3/sec stimuli to the right median nerve at the wrist (Figs. 5–15C and D) revealed a typical myas-

thenic response (50% decline of the evoked response). This fatigue was reversed with intravenous edrophonium.
   B. *SUMMARY OF FINDINGS AND CLINICAL SIGNIFICANCE.* 50% decline of the evoked response on repetitive stimulation of the median nerve. These findings are typical of myasthenia gravis.

VI. COMMENT (Cases 16 and 17). The electromyogram in Case 16 was entirely normal except for diminished recruitment on maximum effort. This is typical of patients with myasthenia gravis, especially with repeated exertion. Repetitive stimulation produced a typical decline of the evoked response, 30% less than the initial twitch height. Nerve conduction velocity values were normal. The reversal of the fatigue response elicited by repetitive stimulation by anticholinesterase medication confirmed the diagnosis of myasthenia gravis. It is important to use repetitive stimuli of 20–30/sec if no fatigue is seen with lower stimulus frequencies. However, normal muscle occasionally may show fatigue above this frequency level and the test becomes painful indeed. A clinically affected muscle should be used for repetitive stimulation because false negative results otherwise can obtain.

Case 18

MYASTHENIC SYNDROME (**Eaton–Lambert**)

I. HISTORY.   This 48-year-old white male was referred for neurologic consultation because of gradual and progressive weakness of the proximal muscles of the extremities. The patient was known to have bronchogenic carcinoma. The tumor was resected partially 1 year prior to consultation. Since that time, he had done reasonably well, without recurrence demonstrable by chest X ray. However, he became weaker and was able to climb stairs only with extreme difficulty and could not rise from a chair without effort.

II. PHYSICAL FINDINGS
   A. *General physical examination.* No abnormalities.
      1. *Mental status and language.* No deficits.
      2. *Cranial nerves.* Intact. There was no ptosis. The extraocular muscle movements were normal. There was no dysphagia or dysarthria.
      3. *Motor.* There was diminished strength of the gluteal muscles and the flexors of the trunk, extensors of the forearm, the deltoids, triceps, and the neck flexors and extensors. However, there was no atrophy. There were rare muscle cramps but the muscles were not tender to palpation.
      4. *Reflexes.* The muscle-stretch reflexes were uniformly diminished. There were no pathological reflexes.
      5. *Coordination.* no deficits
      6. *Sensation.* normal

III. LABORATORY DATA.   Chest X ray revealed evidence of previous surgery but no recurrence of malignancy. Liver function tests were all within normal limits. CBC, urinalysis, and upper GI and lower GI X rays likewise were normal. X rays of the spine were unremarkable. Spinal fluid examination revealed a protein of 22 mg%, no cells, negative serology, and normal electro-phoretic pattern. A muscle biopsy was recommended but not performed. Serum enzymes—including LDH, CPK, and SGOT—were all within normal limits.

IV. CLINICAL IMPRESSION.   Myasthenic syndrome (Eaton–Lambert syn-drome).

V. ENM
A. *NERVE STIMULATION STUDIES (NSS):*

Nerve	LATENCY (msec)				NCV (m/sec)	
	Motor		Sensory			
		N		N		N
R Ulnar	3.0	2.3-3.4			54.5	49-66
R Median	4.4	2.7-4.2			57.4	48-68

B. *ELECTROMYOGRAPHY (EMG).*

L or R	MUSCLE	INSERTION ACTIVITY	POTENTIALS AT REST			MOTOR UNIT POTENTIALS (MUP)				
						Individual MUP			Interference	
			Fib	Pos Waves	Fas	dur (msec)	amp (mV)	% poly-phasic	Pat	amp (mV)
R	Vastus intermedius	N	0	0	0	2-5	2	Inc	3+	4
R	Tibialis anterior	N	0	0	0	5	1.5	Inc	3+	3

C. *SPECIAL STUDIES.*   Repetitive stimulation of the ulnar nerve at 3/sec produced 30% decay of the evoked response from the right hypothenar muscles; at 30/sec, there was 50% facilitation (Fig. 5–16).

D. *SUMMARY OF FINDINGS AND CLINICAL SIGNIFICANCE.   NSS.* Normal conduction studies. Repetitive stimulation at low frequency pro-duced decline of the compound-muscle-action potential, whereas facilita-tion was produced at higher frequencies. *EMG:* Increased number of poly-phasic MUPs seen in both muscles tested.

VI. COMMENT.   Electromyographic and NCV studies were normal except for several areas in which short-duration MUPs were observed. Although this is compatible with a myopathic process, it is not diagnostic. The most significant result was obtained with repetitive stimulation. At 3/sec, a significant decline of the evoked response was produced. At 30/sec, a marked facilitation of the evoked response occurred.

When performing these tests, it is most important to keep the tested hand firmly fixed, because shortening the muscle beneath fixed electrodes allows the motor end-plate region to move relative to the latter. This may produce a false–positive facilitation response. However, the result was significant in the

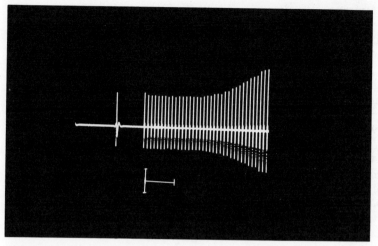

Fig. 5–16. Case 18. Neuromyal junction. Myasthenic syndrome (Eaton–Lambert). Stimulation of the right ulnar nerve with 30/second stimuli, recording from the abductor digiti quinti. 50% facilitation of the evoked response was produced. Calibration: 2 mV, 500 msec.

present case and the diagnosis of Eaton–Lambert syndrome was confirmed. Unfortunately, the patient was lost to follow-up so that the suspicion of recurrent bronchogenic carcinoma could not be verified.

NEUROMYOPATHY

Case 19

POLYMYOSITIS

I. HISTORY.   A 34-year-old black male was admitted to the hospital complaining of generalized weakness. He was well until 6 months previously when, while working as a garbage collector, he slipped while picking up a heavy load. Within 2 weeks, he began to notice that he could not lift heavy objects above his head. Within 2 months, the weakness increased in severity to the point that he was unable to handle heavy objects at all. He had increasing difficulty walking and climbing stairs, and could not rise to his feet after squatting. Reduction in the size of the shoulder muscles was observed. Treatment with steroid drugs produced some improvement so that he again was able to walk and to raise his arms above his head. Treatment was stopped after 1½ months for economic reasons. He remained about the same for some time. He denied any history of pyrexia, arthralgia, or myalgia.

Four months prior to admission, he was found to have marked shoulder girdle atrophy and proximal muscle wasting of the upper and lower extremities. The clinical impression at that time was "muscular dystrophy." Serum glutamic oxalacetic transaminase values varied between 136 and 250 units (normal = < 40 units) Serum glutamic pyruvic transaminase levels ranged between 114 and 220 units. Lactic dehydrogenase measurements ranged between 1680 and 2120 units (normal = < 500 units). Blood count was normal; ESR, 22 mm/hour. X rays of the chest, skull, cervical spine, pelvis, lower gastrointestinal tract, and gall bladder were normal, as was an intravenous pyelogram. ECG also was normal. Muscle biopsy (Fig. 5–17A) was reported as "degenerative muscle changes compatible with polymyositis." There was no family history of myopathy or nervous system disease.

II. PHYSICAL FINDINGS
   A. *General physical examination.* The radial pulse was normal and regular. The blood pressure was normal and the patient was afebrile.
   B. *Neurologic examination*
      1. *Mental status and language.* Normal.
      2. *Cranial nerves.* There was slight bilateral facial weakness but no other deficits.
      3. *Motor.* There was marked weakness in the shoulder girdle muscles bilaterally, with particular wasting of the deltoid muscles (Figs. 5–17B and C). There was also some atrophy and weakness bilaterally of the trapezeii as well as the sternocleidomastoid, biceps (Fig. 5–17D), and triceps muscles. There was minimal wasting of the muscles of the thenar and hypothenar eminences bilaterally. In the lower extremities, there was striking weakness of the proximal musculature, primarily the gluteii and the hamstrings. He had a typical Trendelenberg gait, swinging his body from side to side. In rising erect from the supine position, he used his arms to climb up his body (Gower's sign). No fasciculations were seen.
      4. *Reflexes.* The muscle-stretch reflexes were diminished uniformly throughout.
      5. *Coordination.* No deficits except where limited by weakness.
      6. *Sensation.* No deficits.

III. LABORATORY DATA.
   Hgb, 18 gm%; Hct, 58.5%; WBC, 4250 (repeat, Hgb, 19.5 gm%; Hct, 63%; WBC, 3700). Bone marrow showed a nonspecific hyperplasia. FBS and BUN were normal. An LE preparation was negative. Protein electrophoresis revealed the following fractions (all in gm%); Alpha 1 globulin, 0.3; alpha 2, 0.7; beta, 0.9; and gamma, 1.9. Serum aldolase, 22 units (normal 3–8 units); creatinine phosphokinase, 3,000 units (normal 0–200 units); lactic dehydrogenase, 880 units on admission, and 330 units two weeks later, (normal, 100–450 units). Urinalysis was normal. X rays of the chest were normal, as was an intravenous pyelogram. Slides of the muscle biopsy were reviewed and found to be consistent with a diagnosis of "chronic polymyositis." *HOSPITAL COURSE.* With the presumptive diagnosis of polymyositis, the patient was placed on 80 mg of prednisolone daily for 5 days, which then was tapered to 60 mg/ day. A program of physiotherapy was started. There was considerable improvement on this regimen.

IV. CLINICAL IMPRESSION.
   Polymyositis.

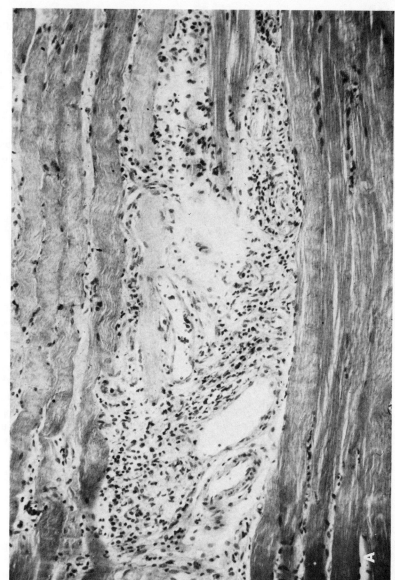

Fig. 5-17 A.

(continued)

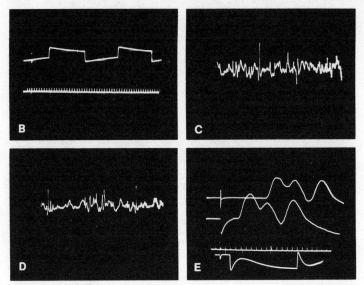

Fig. 5–17. Case 19. Neuromyopathy: Polymyositis. **A.** Muscle biopsy. Focal lymphocytic and mononuclear infiltrate in perivascular adventitial and interstitial connective tissue. Adjacent muscle fibers undergoing degenerative changes. (H&E × 1130). **B.** Calibration for C and D: 20 μV, 1 msec/division. **C.** MUP on maximal voluntary effort. Monopolar recording from right deltoid. **D.** MUP on maximal voluntary contraction: Monopolar recording from right biceps. **E.** Motor NCV, right median nerve:

	d	t
1	340	8.7
2	65	3.2
3	275	5.5

$$V = \frac{275}{5.5} = 50.0 \text{ m/sec.}$$

V. ENM
A. *NERVE STIMULATION STUDIES (NSS).*

		LATENCY (msec)			NCV (m/sec)	
	Nerve	Motor		Sensory		
			N		N		N
R	Median	3.2	2.7-4.2			50.0	48-68
R	Peroneal	4.0	3.7-6.1			44.0	44-58

B. *ELECTROMYOGRAPHY (EMG).*

L or R	MUSCLE	INSERTION ACTIVITY	POTENTIALS AT REST			MOTOR UNIT POTENTIALS (MUP)				
						Individual MUP			Interference	
			Fib	Pos Waves	Fas	dur (msec)	amp (mV)	% poly-phasic	Pat	amp (mV)
R	Deltoid	I	1+	1+	0	1-8	1	N	3+	2
R	Biceps brachii	I	1+	0	0	1-8	1	N	3+	2
R	First dorsal interosseus	I	0	0	0	5-10	5	N	2+	5
R	Quadriceps	I	1+	0	0	2-8	1	N	3+	2
R	Tibialis anterior	I	1+	0	0	2-8	1	N	3+	2
R	Gastrocnemius	I	1+	0	0	2-8	1	N	3+	2

C. *SUMMARY OF FINDINGS AND CLINICAL SIGNIFICANCE. NSS.* Normal. *EMG.* A few fibrillations were seen in most muscles tested. Insertion activity generally was increased. MUPs were of short duration and the interference pattern was full.

These findings are compatible with a myopathic disorder. The presence of fibrillations suggests an inflammatory myopathy.

VI. COMMENT. The EMG findings are typical of those seen in myopathy, namely, numerous MUPs of low amplitude and short duration. The positive sharp waves and fibrillation potentials noted are more typical of an inflammatory myopathy (such as polymyositis) than muscular dystrophy, where electrical silence at rest is the rule. The fibrillation potentials detected in some muscles must be distinguished from small, "sharp" MUPs which are seen with minimal voluntary contraction in diseases of muscle. Here the examiner is dependent on his skill in securing and determining complete voluntary relaxation. The normal NCV values (Fig. 5–17E) confirmed the absence of significant neuropathy. Sampling of several muscles showed the process to be more severe proximally than distally, a finding consonant with a myopathy rather than neurogenic disorder. In this case, the clinical findings, laboratory data, muscle biopsy study, and ENM results all were consistent with the diagnosis of polymyositis.

Case 20

SCLERODERMA

I. HISTORY. This 39-year-old schoolteacher complained of muscle weakness. It began in the thigh muscles 6 years prior to examination. Subsequently she developed trouble climbing stairs and running. There was no family history of a similar ailment. For the past 6–8 years, she had been taking pills for Raynauds's disease, but without relief.

II. PHYSICAL FINDINGS
A. *General physical examination.* There was a discrete reddened, slightly raised rash scattered over the chest, face, and arms.

B. *Neurologic Examination*
1. *Mental status and language.* Normal.
2. *Cranial nerves.* No deficits.
3. *Motor.* The patient had a slow but normal gait. Gower's sign was positive. There was weakness of the proximal muscles of the lower extremities and, to a slight degree, in the upper extremities.
4. *Reflexes.* The muscle-stretch reflexes were diminished throughout. Superficial abdominal reflexes were normal.
5. *Coordination.* No deficits.
6. *Sensation.* No deficits.

III. LABORATORY DATA.   A muscle biopsy (Fig. 5–18A) was considered to be "myopathic," consistent with polymyositis. At about this time, a skin biopsy (Fig. 5–18B) was interpreted as scleroderma. She was placed on prednisone, high-alternate-day doses. This was reduced gradually to maintenance levels. Muscle strength improved and she has continued to function satisfactorily.

IV. CLINICAL IMPRESSION.   Scleroderma with myopathy.

V(a). ENM (First study)
A. *NERVE STIMULATION STUDIES (NSS).*

	Nerve	LATENCY (msec)				NCV (m/sec)	
		Motor		Sensory			
			N		N		N
R	Ulnar	2.3	2.3-3.4	2.9	2.1-3.0	66.2	49-66
R	Median	3.1	2.7-4.2	3.1	2.3-3.2	57.2	48-68
R	Peroneal	3.8	3.7-6.1			51.2	44-58
R	Posterior Tibial	4.8	4.2-6.7			49.3	42-55
R	Sural (7cm)			2.3	1.2-2.5		
R	Sural (14cm)			3.8	3.0-4.0		
R	Sural (21cm)			5.0	5.3-8.8		

Fig. 5–18.   Case 20. Scleroderma. **A.** Muscle biopsy. Degeneration of muscle fibers with replacement by collagenous fibers. (Trichrome, × 125). **B.** Biopsy of skin. Thickened degenerative collagenous fibers can be seen at the left, accompanied by lymphocytic and mononuclear infiltrates. Focal calcific deposits with multi-nucleated giant cells are also present (H&E, × 500). Courtesy of Dr. E. R. Ross.

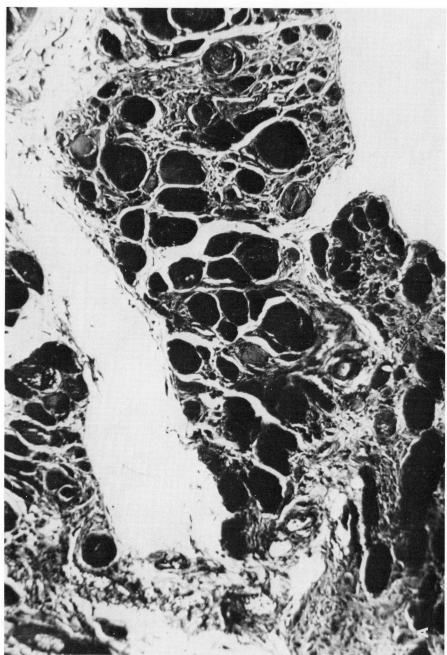

Fig. 5–18 A.

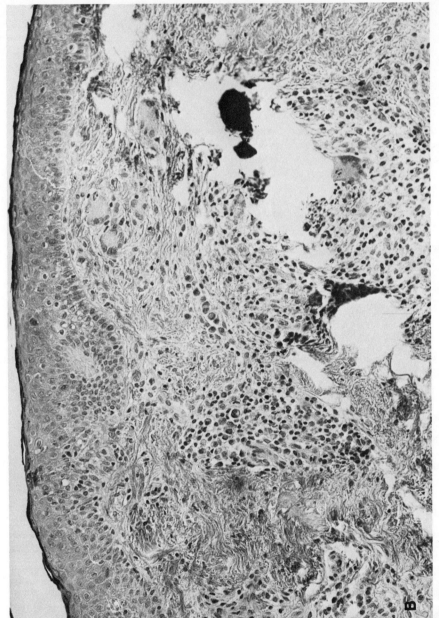

Fig. 5–18 B.

B. *ELECTROMYOGRAPHY (EMG).*

L or R	MUSCLE	INSERTION ACTIVITY	POTENTIALS AT REST			MOTOR UNIT POTENTIALS (MUP)				
						Individual MUP			Interference	
			Fib	Pos Waves	Fas	dur (msec)	amp (mV)	% poly-phasic	Pat	amp (mV)
R	Gastrocnemius	N	0	0	0	1-2	.5-1	N	3+	1
R	Extensor digitorum brevis	N	0	0	0	5-8	.5-1	N	3+	1
R	Vastus medialis	N	0	0	0	5-8	.5-1	N	3r	1
R	Vastus intermedius	N	2+	2+	0	5-8	1-2	N	3+	2
R	Abductor magnus	N	1+	1+	0	1-2	1-2	N	3+	1
R	Vastus lateralis	M II	2+	2+	0	1-2	1-2	N	3+	1
L	Vastus intermedius	N	2+	2+	0	1-2	1-2	N	3+	1
R	Deltoid	N	1+	0	0	1-2	1-2	N	3+	1
R	Brachioradialis	N	0	0	0	1-2	1-2	N	3+	1
R	Supraspinatus	N	0	0	0	1-2	1-2	N	3+	1

C. *SUMMARY OF FINDINGS AND CLINICAL SIGNIFICANCE. NSS.*
Normal. *EMG.* Fibrillations were found in several muscles. In some muscles, MUPs were of short duration and low amplitude. These changes were more marked proximally than distally.

These findings are compatible with a proximal myopathy.

V.(b). ENM (Second study, 6 months later)
A. *NERVE STIMULATION STUDIES (NSS).*

Nerve	LATENCY (msec)				NCV (m/sec)	
	Motor		Sensory			
		N		N		N
R Ulnar	3.4	2.3-3.4	2.9	2.1-3.0	58.4	49-66
R Median	2.3	2.7-4.2	3.1	2.3-3.2	57.9	48-68
R Peroneal	3.9	3.7-6.1			50.0	44-58
R Posterior Tibial	5.7	4.2-6.7			49.3	42-55
R Sural (7cm)			2.3	1.2-2.5		
R Sural (14 cm)			3.8	3.0-4.0		
R Sural (21 cm)			5.0	5.3-8.8		

B. *ELECTROMYOGRAPHY (EMG).*

L or R	MUSCLE	INSERTION ACTIVITY	POTENTIALS AT REST			MOTOR UNIT POTENTIALS (MUP)				
						Individual MUP			Interference	
			Fib	Pos Waves	Fas	dur (msec)	amp (mV)	% poly-phasic	Pat	amp (mV)
R	Tibialis anterior	N	0	0	0	1-2	1	N	3+	1
R	Gastrocnemius	N	0	0	0	1-2	1	N	3+	1
R	Extensor digitarum brevis	M II	0	0	0	1-2	1	N	3+	1
R	Quadriceps femoris	M II	0	0	0	1-2	1	N	3+	1
R	Deltoid	N	0	0	0	1-2	2-3	N	3+	3

C. *SUMMARY OF FINDINGS AND CLINICAL SIGNIFICANCE.*

NSS. Normal. *EMG.* MUPs were of low amplitude and accompanied by type II myotonic discharges.

These findings are consistent with a myopathic process; the presence of type II myotonic discharges with the other findings suggests an inflammatory myopathy.

V(c). **ENM** (Third study, one year later)

A. *NERVE STIMULATION STUDIES (NSS).*

Nerve	LATENCY (msec)				NCV (m/sec)	
	Motor		Sensory			
		N		N		N
R Ulnar	2.1	2.3-3.4	3.3	2.1-3.0	64.0	49-66
R Median	3.3	2.7-4.2	2.9	2.3-3.2	56.8	48-68
R Peroneal	6.0	3.7-6.1			46.8	44-58
R Posterior Tibial	3.3	4.2-6.7			49.4	42-55

B. *ELECTROMYOGRAPHY (EMG).*

L or R	MUSCLE	INSERTION ACTIVITY	POTENTIALS AT REST			MOTOR UNIT POTENTIALS (MUP)				
						Individual MUP			Interference	
			Fib	Pos Waves	Fas	dur (msec)	amp (mV)	% poly-phasic	Pat	amp (mV)
R	Tibialis anterior	N	0	0	0	1-2	1	N	3+	1
R	Gastrocnemius	N	0	0	0	1-2	1	N	3+	1
R	Extensor digitorum brevis	N	0	0	0	1-2	1	N	3+	1
R	Vastus medialis	N	0	0	0	1-2	1	N	3+	1
R	First dorsal interosseus	N	0	0	0	1-2	1	N	3+	1
R	Brachioradialis	N	0	0	0	1-2	1	N	3+	1
R	Deltoid	N	0	0	0	1-2	1	N	3+	1

C. *SUMMARY OF FINDINGS AND CLINICAL SIGNIFICANCE. NSS.* Normal. *EMG.* Some MUPs were of slightly low amplitude but less typically myopathic than previous studies.

These findings represent an improvement over previous examinations.

VI. COMMENT. The initial study indicated normal motor and sensory NCV studies in the presence of abnormal EMG potentials: fibrillations and positive waves. There were distinct alterations in the MUPs: small, sharp potentials, diffuse in distribution. Myotonic discharges (type II) also were observed. Such changes suggest the locus of pathology at the muscular level. The diagnosis of an inflammatory myopathy associated with scleroderma was made from the muscle and skin biopsies coupled with the ENM findings. Repeat ENM studies at 6-month intervals indicated an improvement of muscle status and confirmed the patient's report concerning function. These studies, in addition to blood chemistries (CPK, sedimentation rate, CBC) provide invaluable assistance in monitoring the course of the disease and therapy. ENM in this instance helped to define the area of pathology and added significantly to the confirmation of etiology.

MYOPATHY

Case 21

PROXIMAL MYOPATHY (Suspect Muscular Dystrophy, Limb-Girdle Type)

I. HISTORY. This 20-year-old white female came to the hospital complaining of continuous discomfort and weakness in both legs. Six years prior to admission, strenuous exercise began to cause aching of the posterior aspect of both thighs and legs. Weakness developed and, by the time of examination, she could climb stairs only by pulling herself up the bannister. Despite these disabilities, she continued working as a bank clerk, a job which involved a great deal of walking and standing. One brother, 25 years of age, had similar pains in his legs, but he was said to have had poliomyelitis.

II. PHYSICAL EXAMINATION
A. *General physical examination.* She was moderately obese and of short stature. The arches of the feet were relatively high and there was suggestive clubbing of the toes.
B. *Neurologic Examination*
1. *Mental status and language.* No deficits.
2. *Cranial nerves.* Within normal limits. There was no sternocleidomastoid or facial weakness.
3. *Motor.* There was neither obvious hypertrophy nor atrophy of muscle, but obesity precluded accurate evaluation. There was definite weakness of the peroneal muscle groups bilaterally, and slight paresis of the quadriceps. Winging of the scapula was noted on both sides.
4. *Reflexes.* The muscle-stretch reflexes were depressed uniformly. Even with reinforcement, there were no pathologic toe signs.

5. *Coordination.* No abnormalities.
6. *Sensation.* No deficits.

III. LABORATORY DATA.   Enzyme studies showed serum glutamic oxalacetic transaminase, 18 units; lactic dehydrogenase, 330 units; FBS, 90 mg %;
sedimentation rate, 0 mm /hour; blood count, normal. Thyroid studies (T3,
T4, and T7) were normal. Spinal puncture revealed a protein of 21 mg %, two
lymphocytes, flat colloidal gold curve, and negative Pandy. X rays of the hips,
knees, and ankles showed no abnormalities. ECG was normal.

IV. CLINICAL IMPRESSION.   Progressive muscular dystrophy, limb–girdle
type.

V. ENM
A. *NERVE STIMULATION STUDIES (NSS).*

Nerve	LATENCY (msec)				NCV (m/sec)	
	Motor		Sensory			
		N		N		N
R Peroneal	6.0	3.7-6.1			51.4	44-58
L Posterior Tibial	6.2	4.2-6.7			50.0	42-55

B. *ELECTROMYOGRAPHY (EMG).*

L or R	MUSCLE	INSERTION ACTIVITY	POTENTIALS AT REST			MOTOR UNIT POTENTIALS (MUP)				
						Individual MUP			Interference	
			Fib	Pos Waves	Fas	dur (msec)	amp (mV)	% poly-phasic	Pat	amp (mV)
R	Deltoid	N	0	0	0	2-3	1	N	3+	2
R	Biceps brachii	N	0	0	0	2-3	1	N	3+	2
L	Deltoid	N	0	0	0	2-3	1	N	3+	2
L	Biceps brachii	N	0	0	0	2-3	1	N	3+	2
R	Quadriceps	N	1+ ?	0	0	2-3	1	N	3+	2
R	Biceps femoris	N	0	0	0	2-3	1	N	3+	2
R	Tibialis anterior	N	0	0	0	2-3	1	N	3+	2
R	Peroneus longus	N	0	0	0	2-3	1	N	3+	2
R	Gastrocnemius	N	0	0	0	2-3	1	N	3+	2
L	Quadriceps	N	0	0	0	2-3	1	N	3+	2
L	Tibialis anterior	N	1+ ?	0	0	2-3	1	N	3+	2
L	Peroneus longus	N	0	0	0	2-3	1	N	3+	2
L	Gastrocnemius	N	2+ ?	0	0	2-3	1	N	3+	2
L	Biceps femoris	N	0	0	0	2-3	1	N	3+	2

C. *SUMMARY OF FINDINGS AND CLINICAL SIGNIFICANCE. NSS.* normal. *EMG.* Scattered fibrillations but no fasciculations were noted in several muscles. MUPs were decreased in amplitude and duration (Fig. 5–19A) but there was a good interference pattern relative to the strength of contraction.

These findings are compatible with a myopathy.

VI. COMMENT: The ENM findings are consistent with a primary myopathy. The few fibrillations seen might suggest a neurogenic disorder were it not for the normal NCV studies and the changes in MUP classic for a myopathy. Inflammatory myopathies especially may give rise to fibrillations, although these may be confused with the dwarfed voluntary potentials seen with minimal effort. Clinical correlation and biopsy usually are required to differentiate a dystrophy from an inflammatory myopathy. In this patient, the history, findings, laboratory data, and ENM picture led to the final diagnosis of dystrophy of the limb–girdle type although enzyme histochemistry, had it been available at the time of evaluation, would have been most helpful. In this case, as in others, some features may be atypical, such as the history of pain, the rare "fibrillations," and the questionable family history, but the differential diagnosis of the myopathies is based on probabilities derived from all available data.

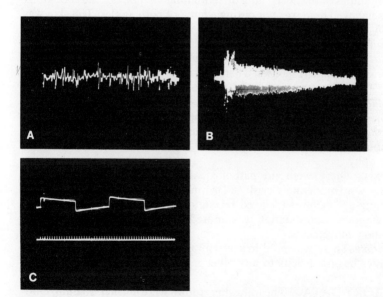

Fig. 5–19. Cases 21 and 22. Myopathy (limb–girdle muscular dystrophy and myotonic dystrophy). **A.** Case 21, limb–girdle muscular dystrophy; MUP recorded from right deltoid, maximum voluntary effort, coaxial electrode. Calibration *(C)* 1 msec/division, 200 μV. **B.** Case 22, myotonia; myotonia evoked on percussion of right opponens pollicis, monopolar electrode. Calibration *(C)* 30 msec/division, 1 mV. **C.** Calibration for *A* and *B*.

Case 22

MYOTONIC DYSTROPHY

I. HISTORY. A 39-year-old housewife came to the clinic complaining of weakness, clumsiness, and lassitude. At age 9 she first found it difficult to walk because she tripped over her own feet. Muscle weakness was slowly progressive but not incapacitating. As recently as 10 years prior to the present evaluation, she was able to perform intricate work in a lock factory. Six years ago, after the last of four pregnancies, she began to notice an inability to relax her grip, and fine finger movements became impaired. In the patient's family, a brother and two cousins were thought to have a similar disorder, and a sister was being treated for hypothyroidism. Of the patient's three daughters, two had myotonia clinically and electromyographically, and all three had some of the features of myotonic dystrophy: posterior cataracts, myopathic facies and speech, and muscle-wasting in the limbs, most prominent in the sternocleidomastoids.

II. PHYSICAL FINDINGS
   A. *General physical examination.* The patient was a rather slow-moving woman with sallow skin and scanty, coarse hair and eyebrows. Her pressure was 90/60 mm Hg, pulse 60/min. Her rectal temperature was 98°F. There were dusty posterior cataracts, the left in the shape of a star. There were no abnormalities of the heart, lung or abdominal viscera, but the abdominal wall was flabby. There was nonpitting edema of both ankles. The skin was dry, scaly, and coarse.
   B. *Neurologic examination*
      1. *Mental status and language.* The patient appeared dull-witted with slow, prolonged, laconic responses. There was no evidence of aphasia or dysarthria.
      2. *Cranial nerves.* There was napkin-ring myotonia of the tongue.
      3. *Motor.* There was bilateral grasp myotonia, but no lid-lag. Occasionally myotonia could be elicited at the thenar eminences. There was slight proximal muscle weakness symmetrical in all four limbs, but there was no atrophy.
      4. *Reflexes.* There were no pathological reflexes. The muscle-stretch reflexes were moderately brisk and symmetrical. There was a suggestion of "hung-up" reflexes (delayed relaxation) at the knees and ankles.
      5. *Coordination.* Coordination was limited by the general slowness of all voluntary movements.
      6. *Sensation.* There was mild loss of vibratory sensation in the lower extremities but no deficits to any other modality.

III. LABORATORY DATA. The following studies were normal: sodium, chloride, potassium, and plasma cortisol. Urinary ketosteroids were 2.9 mg/24 hours (normal 15–16); urinary ketogenic steroids, 5.9 mg/24 hours (normal 7–18). PBI was 1 mcgm%. RAI uptake after 24 hours was 1.4%; after 24 hours, 1.0%. The RAI uptake after TSH stimulation was 2% after 24 hours; cholesterol, 380 mg%. The ECG showed a low-voltage pattern in all leads with premature ventricular and atrial contractions. A chest X ray was unremarkable. Skull X ray demonstrated hyperostosis frontalis interna and a small sella turcica. A muscle biopsy from the left calf revealed irregular hypertrophy and atrophy of scattered muscle fibers with increased fibroadipose connective tissue. In some muscle fibers, a central accumulation of nuclei could be seen. Many fibers showed vacuolization and hyalinization. These findings were considered compatible with a diagnosis of muscular dystrophy. *CLINICAL COURSE.* Treatment with thyroid extract daily produced gradual improvement in mentation, general appearance, and vigor. The myotonia lessened, but did not disappear.

IV. CLINICAL IMPRESSION. 1) Myotonic dystrophy. 2) Hypothyroidism (myxedema).

V. ENM
   A. *ELECTROMYOGRAPHY (EMG).*

L or R	MUSCLE	INSERTION ACTIVITY	POTENTIALS AT REST			MOTOR UNIT POTENTIALS (MUP)				
						Individual MUP			Interference	
			Fib	Pos Waves	Fas	dur (msec)	amp (mV)	% poly-phasic	Pat	amp (mV)
L	Deltoid	N	0	0	0	5-8	1-2	N	3+	2
L	Brachiaradialis	M I	1+ ?	0	0	5-8	1-2	N	3+	2
L	First dorsal interosseus	M I	1+ ?	0	0	5-8	1-2	N	3+	2
R	Opponens pollicis	M I	1+ ?	0	0	5-8	1-2	N	3+	2

   B. *SUMMARY OF FINDINGS AND CLINICAL SIGNIFICANCE. EMG.*
   On needle insertion, type I myotonic potentials were noted in all muscles except the left deltoid (Fig. 5–19B). Potentials resembling fibrillations were scattered in most muscles tested. MUPs were relatively normal in duration and amplitude.
   These findings are compatible with a diagnosis of myotonia. No clear-cut myopathic pattern was noted, but the fibrillation-like potentials may be small motor units. Further EMG study is recommended if clinically warranted.

VI. COMMENT.   The clinical findings of myotonia (grasp and percussion) were confirmed electromyographically by the type I myotonic discharges noted on electrode insertion, during and after voluntary effort, and on percussion of the muscle. The pattern was usually brief and decrescendo, typical of myotonic discharges associated with clinically manifest myotonia. The rare fibrillations observed are consistent with the diagnosis but also may be related to the hypothyroid state (neuropathy with denervation) or may represent a few myopathic MUPs. However, the latter were noted to be within normal limits during requested voluntary effort. The myopathic pattern, however, may appear in muscles other than those demonstrating myotonic discharges. Thus the electromyographer suggested a follow-up EMG study to evaluate these possibilities properly.
   The "dive bomber" (type I) myotonic discharges need to be recognized as distinct from type II (bizarre high-frequency potentials, etc.).

Case 23

TYPE II MUSCLE FIBER ATROPHY

I. HISTORY.   This 5-year-old boy was referred by a urologist because of intermittent bowel and bladder incontinence. His mother noted that he tired easily and had a poor appetite. He had been hospitalized recently for a urinary tract infection. He was said to have been small at the time of birth but not under the minimum weight. He is one of six children and none of the others have had similar difficulty. He was born with pyloric stenosis which was corrected surgically.

II. PHYSICAL FINDINGS
   A. *General physical examination.* He was thin and small for his age (weight 30 pounds). He appeared to be about the size of a 3-year-old.
   B. *Neurologic examination*
      1. *Mental status and language.* No deficits.
      2. *Cranial nerves.* No abnormalities.
      3. *Motor.* All muscles were small, and strength was diminished moderately, especially in the lower extremities.
      4. *Reflexes.* No abnormalities.
      5. *Coordination.* No deficits.
      6. *Sensation.* Normal.

III. LABORATORY DATA.   Routine laboratory studies, including CBC, sedimentation rate, SMA–12, and X rays of the chest were within normal limits. A muscle biopsy of the right quadriceps femoris (fig. 5–20A) revealed decreased numbers of type II fibers.

IV. CLINICAL IMPRESSION.   Type II muscle fiber atrophy.

V. ENM
   A. *NERVE STIMULATION STUDIES (NSS).*

Nerve	LATENCY (msec)				NCV (m/sec)	
	Motor		Sensory			
		N		N		N
R Median	2.1	2.3-3.4	2.0		48.0	48-68
R Peroneal	2.4	3.7-6.1			53.8	44-58

   B. *ELECTROMYOGRAPHY (EMG).*

L or R	MUSCLE	INSERTION ACTIVITY	POTENTIALS AT REST			MOTOR UNIT POTENTIALS (MUP)				
						Individual MUP			Interference	
			Fib	Pos Waves	Fas	dur (msec)	amp (mV)	% poly-phasic	Pat	amp (mV)
R	Tibialis anterior	N	0	0	0	1-2	.2-.5	N	1+	.5-1
R	Gastrocnemius	N	0	0	0	1-2	.2-.5	N	1+	.5-1
R	Biceps brachii	N	0	0	0	1-2	.2-.5	N	1+	.5-1

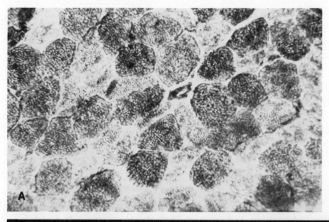

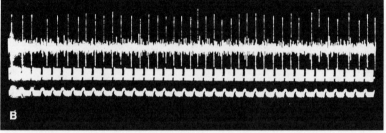

Fig. 5–20. Case 23. Type II muscle fiber atrophy. **A.** Muscle biopsy, right quadriceps muscle, DPNH stain. Note atrophy of type II fibers (light staining). **B.** EMG from right biceps. Monopolar needle electrode. Maximum recruitment. Calibration: 100 μV.

C. *SPECIAL STUDIES.* No decline of the evoked response on repetitive stimulation of the median nerve with rates of 10, 20, and 30/sec.

D. *SUMMARY OF FINDINGS AND CLINICAL SIGNIFICANCE. NSS.* Normal. *EMG.* MUPs were of short duration and low amplitude, with markedly reduced interference pattern (Fig. 5–20B). *Repetitive stimulation study.* No decline of the evoked response on stimulation of the median nerve.

    While these findings are not specific, they suggest the possibility of a myopathy affecting primarily type II fibers.

VI. COMMENT. This patient was brought to the attention of the neurologist by a urologist who was concerned about a possible neurologic basis of the bladder problem. With the history of fatigability and small stature, an ENM was indicated. The ENM findings showed normal NCV and no decremental response on repetitive stimulation. In addition to small motor units, the striking finding of an abnormal interference pattern prompted further study. Laboratory studies, including CPK, Aldolase, and SGOT, were within normal limits. The muscle fibers were generally small (20–30μ). The type II fibers were small and reduced in number. More immature fibers were present than could be accounted for by the age of the patient. ENM was instrumental in the delineation of this rare disorder.

ENM PROBLEM-SOLVING EXERCISES

Cases 24–29 are ENM problem-solving exercises. In each case, the ENM findings will be presented first. On subsequent pages will be found 1) the examiner's analysis of the record, 2) the clinical correlation, and 3) the history, clinical findings, laboratory data, and clinical impression. Thus, the reader has an opportunity to form his own conclusions from available ENM data before proceding to the final formulation.

Case 24.

ENM EXERCISE #1.

I. ENM
  A. *NERVE STIMULATION STUDIES (NSS).*

Nerve	LATENCY (msec)		Sensory		NCV (m/sec)	
	Motor	N		N		N
L Peroneal	3.4	3.7-6.1			46.8	44-58
L Posterior Tibial	5.8	4.2-6.7			43.2	42-55

  B. *ELECTROMYOGRAPHY (EMG).*

L or R	MUSCLE	INSERTION ACTIVITY	POTENTIALS AT REST			MOTOR UNIT POTENTIALS (MUP)				
						Individual MUP			Interference	
			Fib	Pos Waves	Fas	dur (msec)	amp (mV)	% poly-phasic	Pat	amp (mV)
L	Tibialis anterior	N	0	0	0	4-5	1	N	3+	1.5
L	Gastrocnemius	N	1+	0	0	3-5	.5-1.5	Inc	2+	1.5
L	Peroneus longus	N	1+	0	0	5-6	.4-2	Inc	1+	1

  C. *SUMMARY OF FINDINGS AND CLINICAL SIGNIFICANCE. NSS.*
  normal. *EMG.* Denervation potentials were noted in the left peroneus longus and gastrocnemius muscles. MUPs were relatively normal except for reduced recruitment in the left peroneus longus muscle.
  These findings are compatible with a denervative process in the L5-S1 distribution on the left.

II. HISTORY.　This 48-year-old white female librarian gave a history of pain in the left calf and left thigh muscles for 6 months prior to examination. On closer questioning, she related that the muscles of the left calf seemed weak and "mushy." There was no history of difficulty with the upper extremities. Past history revealed hypothyroidism for 25 years; thyroid replacement therapy had been instituted 12 years ago. A cholecystectomy had been performed 18 months prior to admission.

III. PHYSICAL FINDINGS
  A. *General physical examination.* There was no tenderness of the paraspinal muscles nor of any area over the back.
  B. *Neurologic examination*
    1. *Mental status and language.* No deficits.
    2. *Cranial nerves.* No abnormalities.
    3. *Motor.* There were no motor deficits, no atrophy, and no fasciculations.
    4. *Reflexes.* The right-ankle jerk was diminished as compared to the left but the knee jerks were equal. Lasegue, Kernig, and FABER tests were all negative.
    5. *Coordination.* No deficits.
    6. *Sensation.* No deficits.

IV. LABORATORY DATA.   X rays of the lumbosacral spine showed narrowing of the intervertebral joint space between L5 and S1. Analysis of the cerebrospinal fluid obtained at the time of myelography was unremarkable with respect to cell count, protein, and serology. A myelogram was performed and showed amputation of the left nerve root sleeve at the interspace between L4 and L5 (fig. 5–21). She was treated conservatively with bed rest and physical therapy. She made a gratifying recovery.

Fig. 5–21. Case 24. Herniated nucleus pulposus. Lumbar myelogram. Amputation of root sleeve at L4–L5 interspace on the left. Courtesy of Dr. E. Palacios.

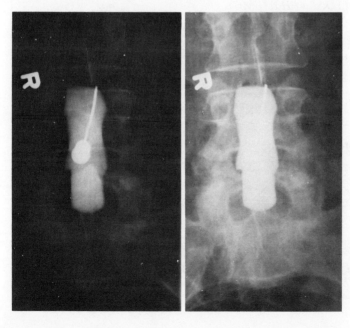

V. CLINICAL IMPRESSION.   Herniated nucleus pulposus, L5–S1 left.

VI. COMMENT.   The normal NCV studies by no means exclude the possibility of a single root lesion, because conduction along fibers from unaffected roots in the same nerve usually produces a normal NCV value. EMG revealed fibrillation (denervation) potentials in the left gastrocnemius and peroneus longus muscles, both of which are innervated by the same nerve root, L5–S1. The tibialis anterior, supplied by the L4–L5 root, was electromyographically normal. In this case, the paraspinal muscles were not examined, a procedure which, in retrospect, might have added additional data to confirm the diagnosis. MUPs were relatively normal, arguing against the anterior horn cell or muscle as the site of involvement. Coupled with the clinical picture, the EMG findings were considered quite compatible with involvement of a single nerve root, in this case a herniated nucleus pulposus, L5–S1, on the left.

Case 25.

ENM EXERCISE #2.

I. ENM
   A. *NERVE STIMULATION STUDIES (NSS).*

		LATENCY (msec)				NCV (m/sec)	
		Motor		Sensory			
	Nerve	N		N			N
R	Ulnar	3.0	2.3-3.4			50.0	49-66
R	Median	5.0	2.7-4.2			49.5	48-68

   B. *ELECTROMYOGRAPHY (EMG).*

L or R	MUSCLE	INSERTION ACTIVITY	POTENTIALS AT REST			MOTOR UNIT POTENTIALS (MUP)				
						Individual MUP			Interference	
			Fib	Pos Waves	Fas	dur (msec)	amp (mV)	% poly-phasic	Pat	amp (mV)
L	Biceps brachii	N	0	0	0	4-8	1-2	N	3+ *	2
R	Deltoid	N	0	0	0	3-6	1.5	N	3+ *	2
L	First dorsal interosseus	N	0	0	0	4-8	1.5	N	3+ *	2
R	First dorsal interosseus	N	0	0	0	5-10	1	N	3+ *	2
L	Tibialis anterior	N	0	0	0	3-6	1	N	3+ *	2
R	Gastrocnemius	N	0	0	0	4-6	2	N	3+ *	2
				* with fatigue on continued effort						

   C. *SPECIAL STUDIES.*   Repetitive stimulation of the right ulnar and median nerves with 20/sec stimuli showed a 33% decline of the evoked response, while 5/sec stimuli produced a maximum of 13% decay (Fig. 5–22).

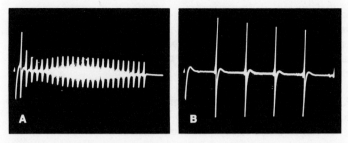

Fig. 5–22. Case 25. **A.** Repetitive stimulation, right ulnar nerve, recording from abductor digiti quinti with stimuli of 20/sec. Calibration, 0.5 mV, 100 msec. **B.** Same as *A,* except stimulus frequency of 5/sec.

gravis.

These findings are compatible with the clinical impression of myasthenia a significant decline of the evoked response.

study. Repetitive stimulation of the right ulnar and median nerves showed prolonged distal latency of right median nerve. NCV normal. *EMG,* normal

D. *SUMMARY OF FINDINGS AND CLINICAL SIGNIFICANCE. NSS.*

II. HISTORY. This 29-year-old white female was admitted through the emergency room because of an acute upper respiratory infection. She was known to have myasthenia gravis for 8 years and had been taking pyridostigmine, 120 mg q.i.d. On the day of admission, she awoke to find it difficult to breathe, swallow, and handle bronchial secretions. She began to have increasing respiratory difficulty and finally lost consciousness. She was taken to the emergency room where she regained consciousness after oxygen and supportive therapy.

Past history includes a thymectomy for a benign thymoma 3 years previously. Following thymectomy, she experienced considerable improvement and remained relatively stable until the day of admission.

III. PHYSICAL FINDINGS
    A. *General physical examination.* The patient was generally weak and debilitated, but with no systemic findings.
    B. *Neurologic examination*
        1. *Mental status and language.* The patient was quite dysarthric and unable to communicate.
        2. *Cranial nerves.* There was bilateral ptosis more marked on the left with dysconjugate extraocular muscle movements. The pupils were equal and reacted to light directly and consensually. Cough was weak and she spoke with a nasal voice. The palate elevated in the midline but the gag reflex was reduced bilaterally.
        3. *Motor.* Flexors of the neck were weak but the extensors were strong. The proximal muscles of the pectoral girdle, including the deltoid and biceps muscles, were weak. Hand grip was relatively strong on both sides. At the time of the examination, respiratory function was adequate: she could count up to 25 on one breath without difficulty.
        4. *Reflexes.* Uniformly diminished and symmetrical; there were no pathological reflexes.

5. *Coordination.* No deficits.

6. *Sensation.* No deficits.

On conservative treatment with intravenous fluids, she recovered gradually and was discharged much improved on 1¼ tablets of neostigmine every 3 hours.

IV. LABORATORY DATA. SMA-12 on admission, unremarkable. White blood count, 6,500, with normal differential. Urinalysis, normal. CPK, 23 units; aldolase, 5.7 units. Chest X ray, unremarkable.

V. CLINICAL IMPRESSION. Myasthenia gravis in exacerbation.

VI. COMMENT. EMG and NCV values were all within normal limits. The prolonged distal latency of the right median nerve is of uncertain significance. The patient's nutritional status was poor, so that a mild neuropathy is a possibility. Repetitive stimulation of the ulnar and median nerves with stimuli of 20/sec produced a definite decline in the amplitude of the evoked response to approximately one-third of the initial (test) potential. This is good evidence of myasthenia, but, without reversal of the fatigue by anticholinesterase medication, a firm diagnosis of myasthenia gravis cannot be made.

Case 26.

ENM EXERCISE #3.

I. ENM

A. *NERVE STIMULATION STUDIES (NSS).*

Nerve	LATENCY (msec)				NCV (m/sec)	
	Motor		Sensory			
		N		N		N
L Median	4.5	2.7-4.2			48.0	48-68

B. *ELECTROMYOGRAPHY (EMG).*

L or R	MUSCLE	INSERTION ACTIVITY	POTENTIALS AT REST			MOTOR UNIT POTENTIALS (MUP)				
						Individual MUP			Interference	
			Fib	Pos Waves	Fas	dur (msec)	amp (mV)	% polyphasic	Pat	amp (mV)
L	Gastrocnemius	N	O	O	O	2-4	.3-.5	N	3+ *	I
L	Tibialis anterior	N	O	O	O	2-5	.3-.6	Inc	3+ *	I
R	Vastus intermedius	N	O	O	O	2-5	.2-.6	N	3+ *	I
R	Deltoid	N	O	O	O	2-4	.2-.5	Inc	3+ *	I
		* Number of MUP increased relative to								
		strength of contraction.								

(clinically muscular dystrophy).

These findings are compatible with a clinical impression of a myopathy relative to the strength of contraction. The number of MUPs was increased increased number of them polyphasic. MUPs generally of short duration and low amplitude, with an tion noted. borderline distal latency of left median nerve. *EMG.* no evidence of denerva- C. *SUMMARY OF FINDINGS AND CLINICAL SIGNIFICANCE.* NSS.

II. HISTORY. When this 10-year-old boy first began to walk at the age of 18 months, his parents noticed that, when arising from a supine position, he seemed to climb up his knees in order to stand. Since that time, his legs became weaker and weaker. At the time of the examination, he could not walk at all, and was confined to a wheelchair. In recent years, the muscles of the upper extremities also had weakened. He had been treated with corticosteroids for 6 years, but to no avail. One brother, age 7, was quite normal and there was no family history of a similar problem.

III. PHYSICAL FINDINGS
  A. *General physical examination.* There was lordosis of the lumbosacral spine.
  B. *Neurologic examination*
    1. *Mental status and language.* No deficits.
    2. *Cranial nerves.* No deficits.
    3. *Motor.* The calves were quite enlarged, and felt "doughy" to palpation (Fig. 5–23A). The muscles in all extremities were quite weak. He "fell through" when the examiner attempted to pick him up under the arms. He could not arise from a supine or sitting position without using his hands to crawl up his thighs (Fig. 5–23 A–C). He barely could stand and hardly could walk.
    4. *Reflexes.* The muscle-stretch reflexes were reasonably active in the upper extremities but were absent even with reinforcement in the lower limbs.
    5. *Coordination.* No deficits.
    6. *Sensation.* No deficits.

IV. LABORATORY DATA. Four years prior to admission, a muscle biopsy of the left gastrocnemius muscle revealed "focal fiber atrophy of skeletal muscle, consistent with muscular dystrophy" (Fig. 5–23C). Another biopsy 2 months later revealed some questionable lymphocytic infiltration, but was considered insufficient for a diagnosis of polymyositis. Serum enzymes: SGOT, 800 units; LDH, 2250 units; CPK, 115 units. Sedimentation rate was within normal limits for his age. Serum electrolytes, normal.

V. CLINICAL IMPRESSION. Pseudohypertrophic muscular dystrophy of Duchenne.

VI. COMMENT. The salient findings of ENM were the abnormalities of the MUPs. They were of low amplitude and short duration, and increased in number relative to the strength of contraction. The number of polyphasic

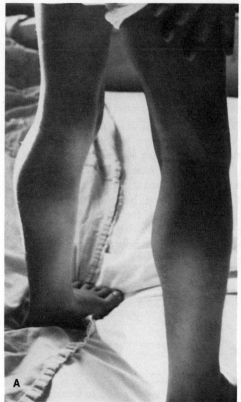
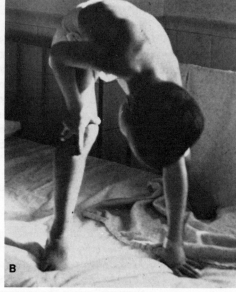

Fig. 5–23. Case 26. Progressive (pseudohypertrophic) muscular dystrophy (Duchenne).
A. Pseudohypertrophy of the calves and atrophy of the thighs. **B.** Illustration of pelvic girdle and paraspinal weakness (Gower's sign). **C.** Muscle biopsy. Marked increase in fibrous connective tissue. There is variation in fiber size with some markedly hypertrophic fibers. Courtesy of Dr. E. R. Ross.

potentials was increased. In the presence of normal NSS, the ENM findings are those of a myopathy. The ENM thus is consistent with the clinical diagnosis of pseudohypertrophic muscular dystrophy.

Case 27.

ENM EXERCISE #4.

I. ENM
   A. *NERVE STIMULATION STUDIES (NSS).*

	Nerve	LATENCY (msec)				NCV (m/sec)	
		Motor		Sensory			
			N		N		N
R	Median	3.6	2.7-4.2			47.0	48-68
R	Peroneal	5.2	3.7-6.1			54.7	44-58

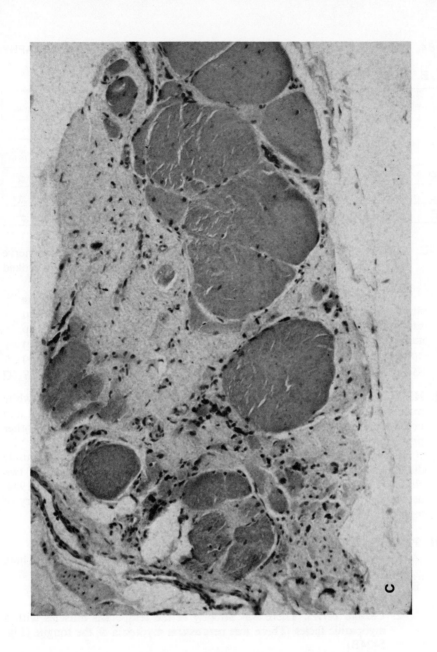

B. *ELECTROMYOGRAPHY (EMG).*

L or R	MUSCLE	INSERTION ACTIVITY	POTENTIALS AT REST			MOTOR UNIT POTENTIALS (MUP)				
						Individual MUP			Interference	
			Fib	Pos Waves	Fas	dur (msec)	amp (mV)	% poly-phasic	Pat	amp (mV)
R	Tibialis anterior	M I	0	0	0	3	2	Inc	3+	2
L	Gastrocnemius	M I	0	0	0	3-5	1.5	Inc	3+	2
R	Opponens pollicis	M I	0	0	0	3-5	0.5	Inc	3+	2

C. *SPECIAL STUDIES.* Repetitive stimulation of the right median nerve with stimuli of 15/ and 20/sec showed no significant decline of the evoked response.

D. *SUMMARY OF FINDINGS AND CLINICAL SIGNIFICANCE.* *NSS.* borderline slowing of NCV of the right median nerve. Repetitive stimulation: no evidence of decline of the evoked response. *EMG.* Type I myotonic discharges were prominent (Fig. 5–24A). Some MUPs were of short duration, and the number of polyphasic potentials was increased. These findings are compatible with the clinical diagnosis of myotonic dystrophy.

II. HISTORY. For at least 1 year prior to examination, this 40-year-old white male had experienced difficulty walking. He began to slap his right foot and noted some weakness of his right hand. However, he was unaware of any other problem.

His father had died of a brain tumor, but there was no history of muscle disease or other neurologic involvement. His own family consisted of two children, both of whom were adopted because of "low sperm count." In 1956, he strained his back while roller skating but there was no other history of injury.

III. PHYSICAL FINDINGS
   A. *General physical examination.* A cataract was found in the left eye. There was definite testicular atrophy.
   B. *Neurologic examination*
      1. *Mental status and language.* No deficits.
      2. *Cranial nerves.* There was atrophy of the temporalis muscles with a myopathic facies. There was percussion myotonia of the tongue (Fig. 5–24B).
      3. *Motor.* There was grasp and percussion myotonia of the hands. The distal musculature of the extremities were markedly atrophic, especially below the knees. He found it impossible to walk on tiptoe or heel on either side even though he could squat or stand up without difficulty. He also could arise from a chair without any effort. There was a marked steppage gait.
      4. *Reflexes.* Within normal limits.
      5. *Coordination.* No deficits.
      6. *Sensation.* No abnormalities.

IV. LABORATORY DATA. None.

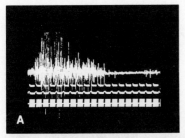

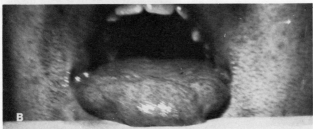

Fig. 5–24. Case 27. Myotonic dystrophy. **A.** Myotonic discharge evoked by percussion. Recorded from the right tibialis anterior; coaxial electrode. Calibration: 100 μV, 100 msec/division.
B. "Napkin-ring" sign elicited by percussion of the tongue using tongue blades (the tongue blade under the tongue has been left in place).

V. CLINICAL IMPRESSION. Myotonic dystrophy.

VI. COMMENT. On NSS the response to repetitive stimulation was normal. The borderline slowing of the right median nerve is of uncertain significance. Measurement of skin temperature in this instance would have been helpful. EMG revealed no fibrillations or fasciculations. Thus there was no evidence for either a neuropathy (peroneal muscular atrophy), as might be suspected from the appearance of his legs, or myasthenia gravis. EMG demonstrated low-amplitude MUPs somewhat diminished in duration, suggesting a myopathic process. The most characteristic feature of the EMG was numerous type I myotonic discharges observed on needle insertion. The diagnosis of myotonic dystrophy, obvious clinically, was confirmed by ENM.

Case 28. ENM EXERCISE #5.

I(a). ENM (First study)
    A. *NERVE STIMULATION STUDIES (NSS).*

Nerve	LATENCY (msec)				NCV (m/sec)	
	Motor		Sensory			
		N		N		N
L Peroneal	NR	3.7-6.1			NR	44-58

B. ELECTROMYOGRAPHY (EMG).

MUSCLE	INSERTION ACTIVITY	Fib	Pos Waves	Fas	dur (msec)	amp (mV)	% poly-phasic	Pat	amp (mV)
		POTENTIALS AT REST			MOTOR UNIT POTENTIALS (MUP) — Individual MUP			Interference	
L Extensor digitorum brevis	I	3+	+1	3+	—	None produced			+
L Tibialis anterior	I	3+	O	3+	—	None produced			+
L Peroneus longus	I	3+	+1	3+	—	None produced			+

C. SPECIAL STUDIES.

EDX. No response from tibialis anterior, peroneus longus, or extensor digitorum brevis with currents of 10–15 ma and 300 msec.

I(b). (Second study, two months later)

A. NERVE STIMULATION STUDIES (NSS).

Nerve	LATENCY (msec) Motor	Sensory	NCV (m/sec)
	N	N	N
L Peroneal (proximal)	3.8	— — —	NR 44–58

(distal latency not obtainable)

B. ELECTROMYOGRAPHY (EMG).

MUSCLE	INSERTION ACTIVITY	Fib	Pos Waves	Fas	dur (msec)	amp (mV)	% poly-phasic	Pat	amp (mV)
		POTENTIALS AT REST			MOTOR UNIT POTENTIALS (MUP) — Individual MUP			Interference	
L Extensor digitorum brevis	I	3+	O	O	—	None produced			+

C. SPECIAL STUDIES.

Continuous S–D curve obtained from the right peroneus longus. Rheobase = 11 ma; chronaxie not obtainable (Fig. 5–25).

D(b). SUMMARY OF FINDINGS AND CLINICAL SIGNIFICANCE (Study #2, two months later).

NSS. Only the proximal latency

D(a). SUMMARY OF FINDINGS AND CLINICAL SIGNIFICANCE.

NSS. No response on stimulation of the peroneal nerve either at the ankle or knee. *EMG.* Numerous denervation potentials noted in all muscles tested as well as numerous fasciculations. No MUPs produced on attempted voluntary movement. *EDX.* No response elicited from either muscle with maximum current.

These findings are compatible with complete denervation of the muscles tested, which implies a complete lesion of the common peroneal nerve. A statement cannot be made as to whether the nerve is or is not in continuity.

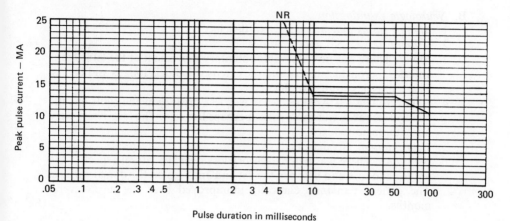

Fig. 5–25. Case 28. Peroneal neuropathy, traumatic. Strength duration curve from the left peroneus longus (from second study, 2 months after initial examination). Rheobase, 11 ma; chronaxie, undetermined.

could be obtained from the left peroneal nerve; this was markedly prolonged. *EMG.* denervation potentials noted in the left extensor digitorum brevis muscle but no MUPs were produced on attempted voluntary movement. *EDX.* rheobase, but not chronaxie, was obtainable from the left peroneus longus muscle. The rheobase was elevated and the S-D curve typical of almost complete denervation.
These findings are compatible with a severe but incomplete lesion of the left common peroneal nerve. The findings are improved compared to the previous study of 2 months ago. The nerve is in continuity.

II. HISTORY. Three months prior to examination, this 15-year-old boy was struck by a car and thrown into a ditch. He sustained a compound fracture of the left leg. X rays revealed a "compound fracture of the left distal tibial epiphysis with 1 inch of intact skin present over the Achilles tendon; fracture of the head of the left fibula with marked displacement." Initial treatment was débridement of the wound and open reduction of the fractures of the distal fibula and distal tibial epiphysis. Internal fixation was accomplished with a screw through the medial malleolus and an intramedullary Rush rod in the fibula. After manipulation and closed reduction of the head of the fibula, X rays revealed excellent reduction of all three fractures. A long leg cast was applied. The cast was removed 2 months later because the leg and foot appeared quite swollen. It was then noted that the boy could not dorsiflex the left foot.

III. PHYSICAL FINDINGS
   A. *General physical examination.* There was a positive Tinel's sign at the left fibular head. There was marked edema and induration of the left lower thigh and also of the lower limb below the knee.

B. *Neurologic examination*

1. *Mental status and language.* No deficits.
2. *Cranial nerves.* No abnormalities.
3. *Motor.* There was no observable voluntary movement of the left tibialis anterior, peroneal muscles and the extensor hallucis longus and brevis. These muscles were atrophic.
4. *Reflexes.* The left Achilles reflex was less brisk than the right but the quadriceps reflex was quite brisk, perhaps less so on the left. There were no pathologic reflexes.
5. *Coordination.* No deficits.
6. *Sensation.* There was patchy sensory loss over the lateral aspect of the left leg and foot and between the 1st and 2nd toes on the dorsal surface. The patient remained clinically unimproved over the next several months.

IV. LABORATORY DATA. None other than above.

V. CLINICAL IMPRESSION. Traumatic lesion of the left common peroneal nerve.

VI. COMMENT. The initial study 3 months after injury revealed no response to stimulation of the left common peroneal nerve. Numerous fasciculations and fibrillations were present in the muscles inervated by this nerve, but no MUPs were produced on attempted voluntary motion. These findings indicated a physiologically complete peroneal nerve lesion; this was confirmed by EDX because no response was obtained with maximum current and duration as the rheobase was sought. Whether the lesion was anatomically as well as physiologically complete could not be determined on the basis of this single test. The patient was asked to return, and did so 2 months later. At that time, fibrillations were still demonstrable in muscles inervated by the left peroneal nerve, but still no MUPs were observed. However, a proximal latency of 28 msec could be obtained from the left peroneal nerve, indicating some recovery (it is also possible that this was a "transmitted" response from other muscles in the anterior compartment). This was confirmed by the strength-duration curve which now showed a rheobase of 11 ma. However, a chronaxy value could not be obtained. Despite the lack of demonstrable clinical improvement, these ENM findings suggested that reinnervation was taking place and surgical intervention therefore was not advised at that time. Instead, physical therapy was continued. Six months later, clinical recovery began in the form of slight abduction of the toes and contraction of the tibialis muscle. However, foot-drop still was present. Subsequently, the patient continued to recover, but his current status is unknown.

In this instance, ENM helped to indicate the continuity of the peroneal nerve and to avoid a needless surgical approach in an attempt to reconstruct a "severed" peroneal nerve at the head of the fibula, which proved to be "physiologically," rather than "anatomically," complete.

Case 29.

ENM EXERCISE #6.

I(a). ENM (First study)
A. *NERVE STIMULATION STUDIES (NSS).*

	Nerve	LATENCY (msec)				NCV (m/sec)	
		Motor		Sensory			
			N		N		N
L	ulnar	3.0	2.3-3.4			65.0	49-66
R	ulnar (surface)						
	to first dorsal interosseus	4.8	3.0-4.5			76.5	49-66
	to Abductor digiti V	3.1	2.3-3.4			52.5	49-66

B. *ELECTROMYOGRAPHY (EMG).*

L or R	MUSCLE	INSERTION ACTIVITY	POTENTIALS AT REST			MOTOR UNIT POTENTIALS (MUP)				
						Individual MUP			Interference	
			Fib	Pos Waves	Fas	dur (msec)	amp (mV)	% poly-phasic	Pat	amp (mV)
R	First dorsal interosseus	N	2+	1+	2+	5-10	1.5	N	3+	4
R	Abductor digiti V	N	0	0	2+	8-10	1.5	N	3+	4
L	First dorsal interosseus	N	0	0	0	5-8	3	N	3+	4

I(b). ENM (Second study, 3 months later.)
A. *NERVE STIMULATION STUDIES (NSS).*

	Nerve	LATENCY (msec)				NCV (m/sec)	
		Motor		Sensory			
			N		N		N
R	Ulnar (surface)						
	to First dorsal interosseus	3.4	3.0-4.5			—	49-66
	to Abductor digiti V	2.2	2.3-3.4			—	49-66
R	Ulnar (needle)						
	to First dorsal interosseus	3.8	3.4-4.5			—	49-66
	to Abductor digiti V	3.8	2.3-3.4			—	49-66

B. *ELECTROMYOGRAPHY (EMG).*

L or R	MUSCLE	INSERTION ACTIVITY	POTENTIALS AT REST			MOTOR UNIT POTENTIALS (MUP)				
						Individual MUP			Interference	
			Fib	Pos Waves	Fas	dur (msec)	amp (mV)	% poly- phasic	Pat	amp (mV)
R	Abductor digiti V	N	3+	2+	0	5-10	1.5	N	2+	2
R	First dorsal interosseus	N	2+	1+	2+	5-7	2	Inc	2+	3

I(c). ENM (Third study, 6 months later)
A. *NERVE STIMULATION STUDIES (NSS).*

Nerve	LATENCY (msec)				NCV (m/sec)	
	Motor		Sensory			
		N		N		N
R Ulnar (surface)						
to First dorsal interosseus	5.0	3.0-4.5			—	49-66
to Abductor digiti V	7.4	2.3-3.4			—	49-66

B. *ELECTROMYOGRAPHY (EMG).*

L or R	MUSCLE	INSERTION ACTIVITY	POTENTIALS AT REST			MOTOR UNIT POTENTIALS (MUP)				
						Individual MUP			Interference	
			Fib	Pos Waves	Fas	dur (msec)	amp (mV)	% poly- phasic	Pat	amp (mV)
R	First dorsal interosseus	N	3+	2+	2+	5-6	2-3	N	1+	3
R	Abductor digiti V	N	0	0	0	6-7	6-8	N	1+	6

I(d). ENM (Fourth study, 6½ months later)
A. *NERVE STIMULATION STUDIES (NSS).*

Nerve	LATENCY (msec)				NCV (m/sec)	
	Motor		Sensory			
		N		N		N
R Median	4.2	2.7-4.2			54.8	48-68
L Ulnar	3.4	2.3-3.4			67.6	49-66
R Ulnar	6.4	2.3-3.4				
axilla-elbow					57.0	50-74
elbow-wrist					38.6	49-66

B(a). *SUMMARY OF FINDINGS AND CLINICAL SIGNIFICANCE* (First study). *NSS.* Prolonged latency to the right first dorsal interosseus muscle, but normal latency to the abductor digiti quinti. Proximal NCV values all normal. *EMG.* Denervation potentials noted in the right first dorsal interosseus muscle. Fasciculations noted in many areas. MUPs normal in duration, but increased in amplitude.

These findings suggest a lesion of the ulnar nerve in the palm of the hand.

B(b). *SUMMARY OF FINDINGS AND CLINICAL SIGNIFICANCE* (Second study, 3 months later). *NSS.* Distal latency of right ulnar nerve prolonged by needle electrode recording, but normal by surface electrodes. *EMG.* Denervation potentials still noted in the muscles supplied by the right ulnar nerve with increased polyphasic potentials. These findings are compatible with a right ulnar nerve lesion, with some reinnervation taking place.

B(c). *SUMMARY OF FINDINGS AND CLINICAL SIGNIFICANCE* (Third study, 6 months later). *NSS.* Prolonged latencies by surface electrodes to both the 1st dorsal interosseus and abductor digiti quinti muscles on the right. *EMG.* Denervation potentials still noted in the right 1st dorsal interosseus muscles. MUPs relatively normal except for reduced interference pattern. These findings have worsened compared to the previous studies 5 months ago:

	Abd. Dig. V.	Normal	1st Dorsal Int.	Normal
Sept.	3.1 msec	2.3–3.4	4.8 msec	3.0–4.5
Dec.	3.8		3.8	
April	7.4		5.0	

Latencies to both muscles are now abnormal.

The patient should return for further study of the more proximal portion of the nerve. These findings are not compatible with a lesion of the ulnar nerve in the palm of the hand.

B(d). *SUMMARY OF FINDINGS AND CLINICAL SIGNIFICANCE* (Fourth study, 6½ months later). *NSS.* Normal latencies and NCV for the right median and left ulnar nerves. The right ulnar nerve shows a prolonged distal latency value. Right ulnar NCV normal from axilla to elbow, but slowed from elbow to wrist.

These findings, coupled with the previous three studies, are compatible with a compression neuropathy of the right ulnar nerve at the elbow.

II. HISTORY. This 45-year-old man complained of numbness and weakness of the right hand for 6 months. Specifically, he noted wasting and weakness of the small muscles of the right hand and some pain and "numbness" in the right shoulder. The symptoms progressed, but he did not complain of cranial nerve involvement or of any difficulty with his legs. A myelogram had been done one month previously; small filling defects at C5–C6 and C6–C7 had been demonstrated. However, these were considered of a minor nature and insufficient to cause his problem. A glucose tolerance test was performed; fasting blood sugar,

102 mg%; ½ hour, 186 mg%; 1 hour, 223 mg%; 2 hours, 120 mg%; 3 hours, 60 mg%; 1+ urinary sugar at 2 hours.

III. PHYSICAL FINDINGS
  A. *General physical examination.* There was a minimal Tinel's sign over the right ulnar nerve at the elbow and also at the wrist.
  B. *Neurologic examination*
    1. *Mental status and language.* No deficits.
    2. *Cranial nerves.* No deficits.
    3. *Motor.* The weakness and atrophy initially were restricted to the right hand, specifically to the 1st dorsal interosseus muscle. The latter was quite atrophic and weak but there were no gross fasciculations. The right abductor digiti quinti was not clinically affected and was quite strong.
    4. *Reflexes.* The muscle-stretch reflexes were brisk and equal. There were no pathologic reflexes.
    5. *Coordination.* No deficits.
    6. *Sensation.* There was minimal loss to pin prick and cotton touch over the tip of the fifth finger of the right hand, but this did not extend into the palm.

IV. LABORATORY DATA.   None.

V. CLINICAL IMPRESSION.   Tardy ulnar palsy (?). Lesion of the deep branch of the ulnar nerve in the palm of the hand (compression neuropathy associated with occupational trauma?).

VI. COMMENT.   The initial study tended to support the diagnosis of mechanical compression of the ulnar nerve in the palm. (latency to the abductor digiti quinti normal, but prolonged to the first dorsal interosseus muscle). However, the difference disappeared over a subsequent period of 3 months and, over the next 6 months, the latency to the abductor digiti quinti was longer than to the first dorsal interosseous muscle. Initially, proximal NCV studies were normal but the final study, 6 months after the first, revealed slowing of the NCV across the right elbow.

  In this case, the EMG revealed denervation in the muscles supplied by the ulnar nerve only on the right side. Specifically, the corresponding left-sided muscles were not affected. Although denervation potentials confirmed the presence of a lower motor neuron lesion, MUPs were normal in duration and amplitude, making the diagnosis of the anterior horn cell as the site of involvement improbable. The possibility of a root syndrome was considered, but the abnormal distal latencies and normal NCVs except for elbow segment argue against this diagnosis.

  The final impression was tardy ulnar palsy, suspect, unverified.

INDEX

INDEX